Research in Criminology

Research in Criminology

Series Editors
Alfred Blumstein
David P. Farrington

David P. Farrington   Lloyd E. Ohlin   James Q. Wilson

Understanding and Controlling Crime

Toward a New Research Strategy

A Report Commissioned by the Justice Program Study Group of the
John D. and Catherine T. MacArthur Foundation

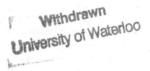

Springer-Verlag
New York Berlin Heidelberg London Paris Tokyo

David P. Farrington
Institute of Criminology
University of Cambridge
Cambridge CB3 9DT, U.K.

Lloyd E. Ohlin
Law School
Harvard University
Cambridge, Massachusetts 02138 U.S.A.

James Q. Wilson
Department of Government
Harvard University
Cambridge, Massachusetts 02138 U.S.A.

Series Editors
Alfred Blumstein
School of Urban and Public Affairs
Carnegie-Mellon University
Pittsburgh, Pennsylvania 15213 U.S.A.

David P. Farrington
Institute of Criminology
University of Cambridge
Cambridge CB3 9DT, U.K.

Library of Congress Cataloging in Publication Data
Farrington, David P.
  Understanding and controlling crime.
  (Research in criminology)
  Bibliography: p.
  Includes index.
  1. Crime prevention—United States. 2. Crime and
criminals—United States. 3. Crime and criminals—
United States—Research. I. Ohlin, Lloyd E.
II. Wilson, James Q. III. Title. IV. Series.
HV7431.F37 1986   364.4'0973   86-11823

Typeset by Publishers Service, Bozeman, Montana.
Printed and bound by R.R. Donnelley & Sons, Harrisonburg, Virginia.
Printed in the United States of America.

9 8 7 6 5 4 3 2 1

ISBN 0-387-96298-0 Springer-Verlag New York Berlin Heidelberg
ISBN 3-540-96298-0 Springer-Verlag Berlin Heidelberg New York

Preface

In 1982 the John D. and Catherine T. MacArthur Foundation created a small committee—the Justice Program Study Group (whose membership is listed at the end of this preface)—and posed to it what can hardly be regarded as an easy question: "What ideas, what concepts, what basic intellectual frameworks are lacking" to understand and to more effectively deal with crime in our society?

Those who are acquainted with the work of the members of the Study Group will appreciate how many divergent views were expressed—divergent to the degree that some of us came to the conclusion that we were not a Study Group at all but rather a group being studied, an odd collection of ancient experimental animals serving some dark purpose of the Foundation. Eventually, however, a surprisingly strong concurrence emerged. We found we were impressed by the extent to which in our discussions we placed heavy reliance on the products of two types of research: first, those few longitudinal studies related to juvenile delinquency and crime that had been pursued in this country and, second, a few experimental studies that had sought to measure the consequences of different official interventions in criminal careers.

These two research strategies had taught us much about crime and its control. Other strategies—case studies, cross-sectional surveys, participant observations, and similar techniques—had indeed been productive, but it was the longitudinal and experimental designs that firmed up the knowledge that the others helped to discover.

We came to the firm conclusion that criminal justice research in the United States has reached a stage at which an increasing investment in more ambitious longitudinal studies is essential. But that was hardly an answer to the question that had been put to us. We had to go further and address the strategy of such studies, and how they should be related to other means of learning about crime and criminals and shaping criminal policy. We needed to confront the considerable obstacles to launching a new research strategy as well as assess what we had already learned, and what we needed to know.

In order to explore these problems, the Justice Program Study Group consulted with 21 scholars in various disciplines, including individuals experienced in longitudinal research. They were asked to prepare brief concept papers on the potential value of and the best design for the next generation of longitudinal studies. Thirteen such papers were prepared.

Together with three consultants—Professor Joseph Adelson of the University of Michigan, Dr. David P. Farrington of the University of Cambridge, and Professor Richard J. Herrnstein of Harvard University, to whom we wish to express our gratitude—the Study Group discussed these 13 papers and then requested the authors of three of them to prepare more fully developed versions for presentation at a conference. These extended statements were prepared by:

1. Delbert S. Elliott, David Huizinga, and Franklyn W. Dunford of the Behavioral Research Institute, University of Colorado
2. Monroe M. Lefkowitz, Long Island University
3. Marvin E. Wolfgang, Deborah J. Denno, Robert M. Figlio, Paul E. Tracy, and Neil A. Weiner of the Center for Studies in Criminology and Criminal Law, University of Pennsylvania

With these three papers providing the raw material for some of our discussions, a conference was then convened in Chicago in June, 1983, to assist the Study Group in its task. More than 50 scholars, researchers, and representatives of government agencies, foundations, and the media attended. Copies of these three papers, which are a rich source of ideas on longitudinal research, may be obtained from the National Criminal Justice Reference Service, 1600 Research Blvd., Rockville, MD 20850.

Two days of vigorous discussion at this conference produced no broad agreement on what the next step in longitudinal studies related to criminality should be, but there was general agreement on the urgent need for such studies. It was probably the fault of the Study Group in its planning for this conference, but there was too much debate about the details of research design and too little attention to the methodological and political realities of laying more secure foundations for such studies and attracting financial support for them. At all events, the conference and the papers prepared in anticipation of the conference provided material that the authors of this book have found invaluable. Indeed, the emphasis during the conference on the great value of combining experiments with longitudinal studies is reflected throughout this book. What we now need is a new research strategy to be launched by a series of relatively small cohort studies of high-risk groups with a variety of experimental treatment modalities attached thereto.

The amplification of that central idea, its explanation and justification, is the purpose of this book. As stated above, that idea no doubt sounds elusive and grossly affected to any reader unacquainted with research in this field, but in the main it is a simple theme: Let us follow the careers of groups of children, youths, and young adults over time, particularly the careers of those who are likely to be involved in crime, in order to try to distinguish those who do become involved from those who do not, to discover which of them persist and which desist, and to learn which treatments seem to work and with whom. This is a well-known strategy in medical research; it is time for its importance to be appreciated and pursued with new vigor in criminological research.

This book makes the case for such research and spells out many of the details by which it could best be pursued. Chapter 1 provides an overview of what we now know about crime and criminals and how we might know more so as to better shape criminal justice policy to our needs. In Chapters 2 and 3, we review in some detail what we have learned from longitudinal and experimental studies in criminology thus far. In Chapters 4 through 7, we explore selected key policy issues to illustrate current deficiencies in the knowledge needed to develop more cost-effective action strategies. In these chapters we consider, respectively, families and schools as targets of prevention measures, theories about the effects of labeling, proposals for reorganizing the juvenile courts, and the effects of imprisonment. Finally, in Chapter 8, we discuss possible research designs and strategies we might now pursue to build firmer ground for our criminal justice policies.

The work of the Study Group was greatly assisted by David R. Ashenhurst, Assistant Director, General Grants Program of the John D. and Catherine T. MacArthur Foundation; it also received encouragement and advice from James M. Furman, Executive Vice-President of the Foundation, and from Edward H. Levi, then a member of its Board of Directors.

Norval Morris

Justice Program Study Group

Daniel Glaser, Professor of Sociology, University of Southern California

Norval Morris, Julius Kreeger Professor of Law and Criminology, University of Chicago

Lloyd E. Ohlin, Touroff-Glueck Professor of Criminal Justice, Emeritus, Law School, Harvard University

Richard B. Ogilvie, Esq., Isham, Lincoln and Beale, Chicago; formerly Governor, State of Illinois

Herbert Wechsler, Director Emeritus, The American Law Institute; Harlan Fiske Stone Professor of Constitutional Law, Emeritus, Columbia University

James Q. Wilson, Henry Lee Shattuck Professor of Government, Harvard University; Professor of Management and Public Affairs, Graduate School of Management, UCLA

Contents

1
The Case for a New Crime Research Strategy: An Overview

Policymakers who wish to put in place new programs to reduce crime, or to expand the scope or effectiveness of programs already in place, will quickly discover that the knowledge necessary to do this responsibly does not exist except in fragmentary and unsatisfactory form. Whether we wish to prevent delinquency or rehabilitate offenders, whether we seek to strengthen families or improve schools, whether we believe that juvenile courts should get tougher or provide better services, we will be forced to admit, if we are honest, that we only have scattered clues and glimmers of hope (and sometimes not even that) on which to base our actions.

This knowledge gap is the largest single impediment to strengthening our society's capacity to cope more effectively with crime. This is the central factual conclusion of the Justice Program Study Group, and it is on the basis of this conclusion that we have chosen to recommend a new research strategy that combines the virtues of longitudinal and experimental methods. In this chapter, we provide an overview of our conclusions and outline a new research strategy. In the chapters that follow, we take up in detail the gaps in our knowledge about crime prevention and the methods that can be used to fill them.

There is nothing new in saying that we do not know enough to mount a well-conceived set of new programs, and there is something a bit lame in calling for more research. In the early 1960s, when crime rates in the United States began their dramatic increase, we knew even less about how to cope with the problem than we do today. Many people were comfortably optimistic about the efficacy of rehabilitation programs; it took a decade or more of research and writing for the realization to sink in that this optimism was misplaced. Others were certain that hiring more police officers and having them engage more frequently in random preventive patrol would cut down on street crime. Again, a decade passed before this certainty was shattered by studies suggesting that feasible changes in levels of preventive patrol would have few or no demonstrable effects on crime rates. Still others believed that the causes of crime could easily be addressed by programs that provided job training, more schooling, and reduced racial segregation. Job-training and job-creation programs flourished; the proportion of young persons staying in school increased; the more obvious forms of racial segregation were overcome. Billions of dollars were spent. Crime continued to rise.

We do not conclude from the history of the last two decades that efforts at crime prevention and criminal rehabilitation are wrong or always doomed to failure, that the police can do nothing about crime, or that efforts to attack the causes of crime are a waste of time. We do conclude that broad-bush, inadequately designed, poorly tested programs are not likely to make much of a difference. We do believe that we have learned a great deal about what does not work, or does not work as easily as we once thought. And we think we have identified those methods of research and experimentation that are best suited for shedding new light on the development of individual differences in criminality and on the strategic opportunities for intervention in that process of development.

When we call for more research, then, it is not because we have learned nothing in the past. On the contrary, as we shall suggest, the best and most useful programs in effect today are based squarely on the best past research. Nor is the call for more research indicative of any desire on our part to postpone action or to underplay the gravity of the problem of crime in contemporary America. Rather, we suggest that the time is ripe for taking a new set of measured steps toward the prevention or reduction of crime and that these new steps can build on efforts already underway. But these steps require, if we are to avoid wasted resources and dashed hopes, a careful specification of the precise points and methods of intervention.

What Do We Know?

We know a great deal about who commits crimes. We know that the typical high-rate offender is a young male who began his aggressive or larcenous activities at an early age, well before the typical boy gets into serious trouble. We know that he comes from a troubled, discordant, low-income family in which one or both parents are likely to have criminal records themselves. We know that the boy has had trouble in school—he created problems for his teachers and does not do well in his studies. On leaving school, often by dropping out, he works at regular jobs only intermittently. Most employers regard him as a poor risk. He experiments with a variety of drugs—alcohol, marijuana, speed, heroin—and becomes a frequent user of whatever drug is most readily available, often switching back and forth among different ones. By the time he is in his late teens, he has had many contacts with the police, but these contacts usually follow no distinctive pattern because the boy has not specialized in any particular kind of crime. He steals cars and purses, burgles homes and robs stores, fights easily when provoked, and may attack viciously even when not provoked. While young, he commits many of his crimes in the company of other young men, though whether this is because they have influenced him to do so or he has simply sought out the company of like-minded friends is not clear. After several arrests, the young man, now in his early twenties, will probably spend a substantial amount of time in jail or prison. The chances are good that not long after he is released from an institution, he will commit more crimes. He runs a high risk of having his life cut short by violent means—the victim of a murder or a fatal car accident.

With these facts in mind, it is not hard to specify a plausible crime control strategy:

Identify these high-risk youngsters at an early age and provide services, counseling, and assistance to their families.
Help them become better students.
Provide assistance and training in finding jobs.
Improve the quality of life in their neighborhoods.
Reduce the availability of dangerous drugs, and provide treatment programs for those persons who abuse such drugs as are available.

But if they commit a serious crime:

Arrest and prosecute them promptly.
Send them to a correctional program that is suited to their temperament and personal history.
While in that program, help them maintain contact with those decent friends and family members whom the offenders cherish.
On release from that program, help them find a job and give them financial and other forms of assistance so that they can try to make a go of it back in society.
If they return to crime after their release, send them to an even more secure correctional institution for an even longer time.

Not only is such a strategy plausible, but many elements of it are being practiced almost everywhere and all elements of it are practiced in some places. But what is plausible might not always be feasible, and what is feasible might not always be valuable. How can families be assisted? Which forms of assistance make a difference and which are wasted efforts? How do you help a rebellious, unmotivated, low-achieving student? What can be done to place a young man with a poor school record and disorderly habits in a worthwhile job? Indeed, how in many inner-city neighborhoods do you find a job for even a competent, well-motivated young man? Which aspects of neighborhood life are worth improving and how do you do it? Does it make a difference who the boy's friends are and, if it does, how can you change those associations? If the youngster likes to drink or take drugs, how do you talk him out of it, especially if all his friends are doing the same thing? If he is arrested early in his criminal career, will this deter him from future crimes or so stigmatize him that he is driven to seek out criminal friends and criminal opportunities? If he is sentenced to some correctional program, which one will be best suited for him and how do we know it will work?

On the basis of past research, scholars and practitioners have been able to describe the typical criminal career with some accuracy. The path-breaking studies of criminal careers by, among others, William and Joan McCord (1959), Sheldon and Eleanor Glueck (1950, 1968), Donald West (1982), Donald West and David Farrington (1973, 1977), and Marvin Wolfgang and colleagues (1972) have taught us to be especially concerned with the small proportion of boys who become very-high-rate offenders. On the basis of this teaching, police officers have formed special units to detect and apprehend high-rate offenders, prosecutors have reorganized their staffs so as to expedite the investigation and prosecution of high-rate and dangerous offenders, judges have been supplied with methods to help them distinguish between low-rate and high-rate offenders, and parole boards have devised prediction scales to help them discriminate between low-rate and high-rate offenders when the boards are deciding whom to release on parole. We believe these research-based changes in criminal justice practice have been cautious, though none is free from criticism. In this and other ways, research has helped society improve its response to crime.

But a great deal remains to be done. For example, if we wish to improve the policy of selectively seeking out high-rate offenders for arrest, prosecution, and incarceration, we need to know much more about who such persons are and how they can be identified. Even then, of course, there will remain some ethical and legal questions about the fairness of a selective policy. But more important, the research that has been so helpful in focusing attention on the high-rate offender has taught us very little, if anything, about how we might prevent a boy from becoming a high-rate offender in the first place. If we could reduce the probability that any given boy who commits one or two offenses will go on to commit 10 or 12, we will have spared society countless victimizations. To do this, we need to learn more about how to prevent the onset of a serious delinquent career and how best to handle the would-be offender in the school system and the active offender in the criminal justice system. We think these things can be learned—not enough, perhaps, to make dramatic reductions in crime, but enough to improve significantly our present policies. At present, we cannot recommend ways to make these improvements because we are at the limits of what can reasonably be inferred from available evidence.

What Do We Need to Know?

Let us review what we know about the correlates of criminality in order to assess which of these are in fact causes of crime and, of course, which might be changed by planned interventions.

THE FAMILY

Almost no one denies that high-rate offenders are likely to come from homes that are cold, discordant, and inconsistent with respect to management of discipline. There is also evidence that such offenders are more likely to come from large, low-income families than from small, higher-income ones. Moreover, some people believe that single-parent homes and abusive parents produce a disproportionate number of offenders, but the evidence on that is not clear.

Let us assume that what has happened in a family does in fact cause, and is not simply an accidental correlate of, delinquency. (As we shall see in a moment, that assumption is not always warranted.) There are at least three different hypotheses that could explain how this causal connection might occur. These include:

1. Economic adversity causes family stress that in turn causes parental discord and (possibly) child abuse. Discord prevents the effective socialization of the child, and abuse teaches him that violence is an approved or useful way of getting what he wants.
2. The parents' temperament (poorly controlled hostility, little regard for the feelings of others, excessive drinking) leads to discord between mother and father, poor or inconsistent child-rearing practices, and unsuccessful employment experiences. The child is inadequately socialized; the marriage founders.
3. The child's temperament (alternately passive and fussy, possibly hyperkinetic, hard to manage) leads to stress in the family, discord between the parents, and the frantic resort to inappropriate child-rearing methods. The child becomes delinquent and the parents seem unable to prevent it. They blame each other for this failure, which intensifies their quarrels and increases the risk of the marriage dissolving.

Obviously, several of these causal patterns may operate simultaneously. But let us assume, for purposes of discussion, that one pattern explains the child's becoming predisposed toward delinquency. Which pattern it is will determine what policies we might wish to endorse, and these policies are likely to differ greatly according to that pattern. Note also that studies that measure the correlation between family circumstances and delinquency cannot uncover the causal pattern; all such studies will simply reaffirm that there is some connection among family adversity, parental discord, weak child-rearing practices, individual temperaments, and early delinquency.

For example, if the first hypothesis is correct, then policies designed to relieve the economic burden on poor families would become important. We might wish to propose the adoption of more comprehensive and effective job-training and job-placement programs or some form of a guaranteed annual income (or negative income tax) or major changes in the amount of and eligibility for welfare and other public assistance programs. This would have to be done carefully. If the benefits are too great, work incentives would be weakened and mothers might find it profitable to remain unmarried and unemployed. But if the benefits are too small, economic adversity would not be reduced sufficiently to prevent acute family stress. Nonetheless, we know where to start.

If the second hypothesis is correct, changing the economic circumstances of the family would have little or no effect on how the child was reared. In this case, economic adversity is not the cause of family stress (though it may contribute to it). Rather, it is the temperament of the mother or father (or perhaps both) that leads to impulsiveness, constant bickering, unpredictable eruptions of hostility or moodiness, and drug or alcohol abuse, and it is these behaviors that lead to both failure in the job market and failure as parents. Psychologists believe that temperament is to some degree inherited; estimates of heritability ordinarily range around 0.25 or 0.30 (Cattell, 1982). And alcoholism has a strong genetic component (Bohman, 1978; Cloninger, Bohman, and Sigvardsson, 1981; Vaillant, 1983). Measures to raise the incomes of such families might succeed, but the behavior of these families would remain pretty much as before. We could instead explore policies that would improve the competence of these parents by teaching them how they might better achieve their own goals by managing their children more effectively, supplementing this with intensive efforts to treat alcoholism or drug abuse. If we cannot design programs that effectively intervene in existing families, we might wish to explore ways of enlarging and improving the provision of foster care for children in at-risk families. The family (or juvenile) court might play a more aggressive role in the early identification of such families. Such programs are not easily conceived or implemented, but if put in place they would address the key factor in the etiology of delinquency.

Now suppose the third hypothesis is correct—that it is the child himself who is in a sense "causing" his own delinquency because he is presenting to otherwise capable and caring parents an especially difficult socialization problem. There is evidence, for example, that low-birth-weight children are inordinately at risk for child abuse because, it seems, such children are relatively passive (they do not reward parents with cooing and smiling), they have difficult temperaments, and are likely to be below normal in intelligence (Belsky, 1980, 1981; Kumar, Anday, Sacks, Ting, and Delivoria-Papadopoulos, 1980). Or the child may be born with minimal brain damage, possibly owing to parental or perinatal stress (such as alcohol or drug abuse by the mother or oxygen deprivation during birth). Or the child may have had a normal birth but be hyperkinetic, so that he is very difficult to control. Improving the competence of the parents might make some difference in how the child is raised, but routine competence may be insufficient. Indeed, family discord may arise because the parents wrongly blame each other (or themselves) for their apparent failures. Should this causal pattern exist, we would want to explore ways of reducing the incidence of prenatal and perinatal stress (by, for example, improving prenatal care, dissuading pregnant women from using alcohol or drugs, and altering diets) and ways of managing hyperkinetic children (by appropriate drug and other therapies).

None of these policies is at all fanciful, though each is difficult and requires careful testing. Increasing family income is politically but not technically difficult; improving parental competence has been successful in some experimental projects (Patterson, Chamberlain, and Reid, 1982); we are learning more all the time about ways of managing difficult children. Some readers may feel that the problem of crime is sufficiently serious, that the prudent course is to try everything at once; but that, we think, is unrealistic. If all were tried simultaneously and the combination produced a good result, we would not know which program was making the difference. Then, if for fiscal or political reasons programs had to be cut, we would not know which could be safely cut. Moreover, each program would be controversial because of cost or incentive effects, because of the degree of intrusiveness into family life, or because medical methods for altering behavior make people worry about the potential for manipulation and the risk of harmful side effects. It would be far better to discover what causal pattern is in fact operating before designing any large-scale effort to alter it. With existing knowledge, we cannot make that judgment.

SCHOOLING

There is little doubt that high-rate delinquents tend to do poorly in school. There is great doubt as to why this should be so. As a result, we cannot be certain what kinds of school programs, if any, would make a lasting difference for a large number of children who seem predisposed to delinquency. Again, there are several alternative hypotheses:

1. Children with mild behavioral problems become labeled as troublemakers in school. As a result, teachers come to have lowered expectations for them, the stigmatized children associate with other troublemakers, and breaking the rules comes to be more satisfying than conforming to adult standards.
2. Children with below-normal levels of intelligence or other learning disabilities find school work frustrating or boring or both. They become restless and take satisfaction in activities—fighting, truancy, rowdiness, sports—for which their cognitive deficits do not disqualify them.
3. Predelinquent children are aggressive and antisocial before they come to school. School may provide them with greater opportunities for mischief and acquaint them with some like-minded friends, but school does not cause their delinquency.

As with family processes, so with school processes: The causal pattern, and hence the appropriate remedial strategy, is unclear. If youngsters become delinquent because they are labeled as troublemakers, then changing teacher expectations and behavior should reduce delinquency. If frustration born of learning difficulties leads to delinquency, then devising better ways to teach and stronger rewards for mastering classroom assignments should reduce the frustration and thus the delinquency. If children have already become overly aggressive and undisciplined before entering school, then schools or preschool programs will have to be created and managed that will, if possible, counteract these predispositions.

As we note in Chapters 3 and 4, there is some experimental evidence suggesting that certain preschool programs may succeed in reducing later delinquency and that schools with a certain ethos and balance of academic talents may reduce delinquency during the school years. These glimmers of hope are worth pursuing, but many questions remain unanswered. We cannot be confident that the reduction is real because (with respect to preschool programs) it has so far only been measured in one or two experimental projects that involve a small number of pupils. Such projects may appear to succeed because the experimenters are able to attract the most talented and dedicated teachers; whether the same treatment would work if applied by less gifted teachers to large numbers of pupils is not clear.

Even if the delinquency-reduction effect of preschool education is real, no one yet knows what it is about the program that produces this effect or for what kinds of children the program is best suited. Does preschool education work because it removes the child from adverse family conditions, or does it work because it supplements and strengthens the well-intentioned efforts of parents to cope with a difficult child? Would preschool education be harmful for children who are thereby removed from a good family, or would such education help all children whatever their family life? Is the key element of the program the cognitive preparation of the child for group activities? Does the program reduce the rate at which any enrolled child will later commit offenses or only the rate at which certain kinds of children (say, those who would otherwise become low-rate offenders) commit future delinquencies?

Many of the same questions can be asked about research showing the desirable effects of attending schools with a certain organizational ethos or character. Is the reduction in delinquency and school misconduct limited to the school-age years, or does it persist after school? Is there a reduction in the serious delinquencies of high-rate offenders or only in the kinds of minor offenses and truancies that are displayed by a very large proportion of all school children? Can a desirable school ethos be created by plan so that children randomly assigned to such a school will show markedly better behavior than similar children assigned to a conventional school?

We seem closer to identifying ways of improving schools than we are to finding methods of improving families, but we are far from knowing how to mount large-scale efforts through the schools and whether, if mounted, they would have a minor or a major effect on later criminality. There have been countless school-based programs tried in the past; the results of most have been dashed hopes. To improve the chances of success, we have to know more precisely what the causal connections are, if any, between schooling and later conduct. We are not much closer to answering that question today than we were 30 years ago.

DRUG ABUSE

High-rate offenders typically are involved with drugs or alcohol abuse. Studies at Rand (Chaiken and Chaiken, 1982) and elsewhere suggest that regular drug abuse is one of the characteristics of the most dangerous offenders. For example, offenders may commit six times as many nondrug crimes when they are using heroin on a daily basis as they would during periods when they are off the drug (Ball, Rosen, Flueck, and Nurco, 1981).

Almost everything we know about persons who are physiologically or psychologically addicted to drugs comes from studying those who are deeply into their addictive behavior and happen to have been arrested or to have volunteered for a treatment program. Such persons are likely to be a quite unrepresentative sample of all those who have experimented with drugs. Because of this, we cannot be confident we know the characteristics of persons who are high-rate users as opposed to casual experimenters or "chippers." There is a sharp disagreement among experts about the effects on high-rate users of a law-enforcement crackdown on drug trafficking. Some argue that such policies reduce the availability of drugs and thus reduce their use; others argue that these policies merely drive up the price of the drugs and thus induce users to commit more crimes to pay for their habits; still others suggest that crackdowns have no discernible effect at all on the supplies available to regular users.

To answer either question requires that we learn more about the individual characteristics of novices and desisters. Efforts to infer what factors predispose some persons to drug use have had to rely, for the most part, on studies of persons already known to be users, and much of that research has been limited to gathering readily available social and demographic data (age, ethnicity, family circumstances) plus, occasionally, psychological profiles. But it is quite possible that there are physiological or biological factors that put some young persons at greater risk for drug abuse than others, just as we already know that there is, to some extent, a genetic basis for the tendency to abuse alcohol. Systematically investigating these and other possibilities is essential if we are to do anything more to prevent drug abuse than mount broad-gauge, ill-focused, and usually untested educational programs designed to persuade young persons to avoid drugs.

EMPLOYMENT

Since high rates of criminality occur disproportionately among people who have low incomes and spotty employment records, it is only natural to assume that poverty and unemployment cause crime. They may, but the case for that connection has not been firmly established; and there exist other possible explanations for this observed connection. For example:

1. People turn to crime because they are unable to find jobs.
2. Certain intellectual and temperamental characteristics (e.g., low verbal aptitude, impulsiveness, little regard for others) may cause some people both to turn to crime and to be unattractive to prospective employers.
3. People who find crime very rewarding (e.g., drug dealers) may reject available jobs and thus be counted as "unemployed."
4. Youngsters raised in neighborhoods where affluent criminals have become role models may not value the benefits of legitimate work.
5. People raised in neighborhoods suffering from chronic shortages of jobs may assume without individually exploring the market that jobs are not available and, hence, training for jobs is pointless (*understanding, 9*).

Though some studies have shown a correlation between crime on the one hand and unemployment, economic recessions, and lowered labor force participation on the other, these correlations are in many cases not strong. Other studies find no such correlation. And where significant correlations do exist, they tell us very little about which of the causal mechanisms listed above, or others that we might imagine, are actually operating. The inconclusive nature of these studies may well result from their relying, with very few exceptions, on aggregate data—that is, on the crime and unemployment rates for entire cities, counties, or states. What is needed are more studies measuring the effects of *individual* experiences in the labor market on *individual* tendencies to commit crime.

Efforts to reduce criminality by experimental interventions designed to supply job training, find employment, and even subsidize ex-offenders looking for employment have so far produced only a few encouraging results (these studies are summarized in Chapter 3). But these programs have generally been directed at adult offenders, ex-convicts, or delinquent school dropouts who are age 18 or older. It may be impossible to intervene successfully this late in the criminal or delinquent career; perhaps starting such programs much sooner, before crime itself has become rewarding, would make a greater difference. Or it may be that the temperamental and cognitive problems of persons who become high-rate offenders cannot be changed significantly by employment and job-training programs. Or it may be that such programs will work, but only if the participants are removed from those neighborhoods that make hustling more attractive than work.

In short, a serious investigation of the connection between crime and work may have to start much earlier in the lives of young men than is commonly supposed. In particular, we may need to know more about the earliest work experiences of youngsters and the relationship between schooling and work. The transition from school to work is poorly understood, especially for those young people who drop out of school early. In studying that connection, we should not begin with the assumption that dropping out of school is always a bad idea. Some persons may benefit from leaving school before graduating, provided they can thereby enter into the discipline of the workplace (Elliott and Voss, 1974). We know too little about the differences among people that affect how entry into the work force is (or is not) accomplished.

JUVENILE COURT

The debate over the role of the juvenile court is a familiar one. Those who think crime can best be reduced by making the penalties for its commission greater want to see the court take seriously the first nontrivial infraction of a youngster by imposing on him some significant penalty (incarceration, mandatory community service, victim restitution) early in the delinquent career in hope that this first short, sharp shock of punishment will deter future and greater misdeeds. If the youngster should persist in criminality, the penalties should be steadily increased, if necessary by transferring him to the jurisdiction of adult court where long sentences can be handed out. Juvenile records should automatically be made available to adult court authorities when the youngster reaches the age of transition. There are studies that suggest that this strategy may work (e.g., Murray and Cox, 1979; Feld, 1981).

Those people who think crime can best be prevented by providing services rather than punishment and by avoiding the stigmatizing effects of early punishment recommend a different strategy. Unless the offense is serious, the child should be diverted from the criminal justice system and into counseling and helping agencies—foster homes, halfway houses, and the like. Juvenile proceedings and records should be confidential and the juvenile record should not automatically follow the child into adulthood. Early punishment does not deter, it merely labels the recipient in a way that is destructive to his self-esteem and exposes him to a greater likelihood of hostile police surveillance. Many delinquents are the product of child abuse and the juvenile court should work to undo the harmful effects of these early experiences. Transferring the juvenile to adult court rarely makes sense. There are studies that seem to support this line of reasoning (Farrington, 1977; Farrington, Osborn, and West, 1978).

The debate is as old as the juvenile court itself. We are under no illusion that research will settle it since what is at stake are not merely facts but also deeply held convictions about the right relationship between the child and society. But the facts are not irrelevant. And they are very much in dispute. Precisely because juvenile records are relatively inaccessible in many jurisdictions, very few studies have followed a group of young persons as they have moved from their first experience with the juvenile authorities to their last and on into the adult system. Because the juvenile system often does not produce statistics equivalent to those produced about adult offenders (even the number of juveniles handled by the court is rarely broken down by type of offense), there are not even many correlational studies of how juvenile courts process young offenders and with what effect.

As a result, we cannot say with confidence that, other things being equal, a delinquent who is punished after his first offense is more or less likely to commit another crime than one who is treated. We only have fragmentary evidence as to the effect—in sentence length and later criminality—of transferring juveniles to adult court. We cannot be certain that adult offenders are sentenced differently when their full juvenile records are known than when they are not.

Moreover, we do not know the consequences of having decriminalized the so-called "status offenses" (i.e., behaviors that, if engaged in by an adult, would not be regarded as criminal). Liberals and conservatives alike in recent years have pressed the states to eliminate such categories as "person in need of supervision" from the offenses dealt with by juvenile courts. But there is some reason to worry about this. First, many persons "in need of supervision" often turn out to be the same persons who are committing delinquent acts. Second, if the juvenile court does not attend, however imperfectly, to the needs of persons needing supervision (runaways, truants, and the like), who will? We recall the enthusiasm which in the 1960s greeted plans to deinstitutionalize mental patients and the dismay that set in during the 1980s when it became evident that the deinstitutionalized patients now made up a large share of the homeless, uncared for by anyone save, occasionally, a sheriff who found space for them in the local jail.

ADULT COURTS AND CORRECTIONS

The issues swirling about the adult criminal justice system are no less obscure. The debate over the purpose of that system—deterrence, incapacitation, rehabilitation, retribution—is a familiar one. Like the debate over the juvenile court, facts alone will not resolve it. But facts will narrow the zone of disagreement by shedding light on the consequences of policy alternatives.

We know more about adult than about juvenile crime and more about adult corrections than juvenile corrections. We have better data for adult than for juvenile offenders on recidivism, the extent of drug and alcohol abuse, and the past employment record. In fact, much of what we know about the nature of criminality has been learned by tracing backwards the careers of arrested adult offenders. But for reasons explained in Chapter 2, these retrospective studies are subject to substantial errors in the accuracy of the offenders' memories and their willingness to be candid. Moreover, retrospective studies do not illuminate the causal sequences by which one circumstance (say, trouble in school) did or did not lead to another (say, trouble in finding a job). And good retrospective studies are few in number. As a result, even for the workings of the adult criminal justice system, much of what we know, about deterrence, for example, comes from cross-sectional or correlational studies that leave the issue of causality rather clouded.

Does imprisonment deter the person imprisoned, or are prisons "schools of crime" that increase the number and enhance the success of subsequent efforts at crime? We have some aggregate studies that shed light on this issue (our best guess is that, on the average, imprisonment makes the offender neither better nor worse) but few that permit us to be very confident about our conclusions. And such studies as do exist tell us only what the effect of imprisonment is *on the average*—none tells us, with much precision, what the effects may be on different kinds of inmates; and hardly any tell us whether *non*imprisonment sanctions (fines, community service, restitution) deter offenders and, if so, what kinds of sanctions, how, and under what circumstances.

The criminal justice system has always been selective about whom it imprisoned. The current debate over "selective incapacitation" is new only in being a debate; the practice is as old as the first trial. For all practical purposes, the issue is not whether the system will be selective (by trying to focus on the most dangerous or the highest-rate offenders) but whether it can be significantly more accurate than chance in identifying those offenders and can do so at an acceptable cost in money and fairness. As we stated at the outset of this chapter, important and sophisticated attempts have been made (by researchers at Rand, among others) to specify the characteristics of high-rate offenders so that they can be identified as early in their careers, and as early in the criminal justice system, as possible. But these studies are retrospective inquiries into the self-reported criminal careers of incarcerated inmates. Not only are they subject to the previously mentioned errors in recall and honesty, but they are likely to be biased by examining only those offenders who happen to be in prison. If one wished to change sentencing policies in order to make more efficient use of scarce prison space by giving prison terms to high-rate offenders, the key issue is what will happen to the crime rate if these decision rules are applied to convicted offenders not now in prison and whose individual offense rates are unknown.

Much the same argument can be made about the current state of our knowledge of rehabilitative techniques. There is no reason to be optimistic as yet about our ability to reduce recidivism rates by plan and for large numbers of offenders. But neither is there reason to believe that no program can ever be effective for anyone. Some experts have argued that the disappointing results of rehabilitative programs arises from failing to see that the desirable effects on some persons are counterbalanced by the undesirable effects on others, giving an average result of "no effect." If different programs are designed for different kinds of offenders, better results, at least in some cases, would be obtained. We do not know whether this conjecture is well founded or not, but we see no reason why it should be dismissed out of hand.

Individual Differences

At least one central theme runs throughout this discussion of what we need to know to improve our ability to prevent crime: The importance of knowing more about *individual differences* among offenders and nonoffenders. The great bulk of policy-relevant research groups offenders together into broad categories, often differentiated (if at all) only by such obvious characteristics as sex, age, race, and official record. But if we wish to reduce the probability of low-rate offenders becoming high-rate offenders, we must develop greater insight into far more subtle differences among individuals and their circumstances. If families differ in the extent to which they produce delinquents, it is not, we think, because such families differ in the age or race of the parents; rather, it is because they differ in the extent to which they form strong bonds of affection with their children, manage effectively the daily routine of socialization and guidance, and cope satisfactorily with both the cognitive and temperamental characteristics of their offspring and the economic and social aspects of their environment. Similarly, if schools differ in their ability to induce reasonable levels of obedience in their pupils, it is not because the schools differ in the age of their buildings or the size of their libraries, but because they differ in the mix of talents among their students and the habits and styles of their teachers.

How Can We Find Out?

Because the design of almost any new crime-reduction policy requires us to choose among equally plausible but competing theories about how individuals respond to the circumstances in which they find themselves, the policymaker's first task is to recognize the need for a research strategy that will guide and test that design. This is especially true if our goal is "primary prevention"—that is, reducing the chances of a given child becoming delinquent in the first place. Uncovering the subtle interaction between individual characteristics and social circumstances requires policy-related research of a sort and on a scale that has not been attempted before.

Some people are ready to acknowledge that we have gaps in our knowledge but argue that they can be filled from the lessons of practical experience. This is misleading. "Practical experience" is itself a form of research; it is an effort to learn by observation. The key question is whether those observations are accurate or inaccurate, systematic or casual, verified or not. Practical experience is an important guide to action, but it is only a guide. To become the basis for a general rule, it must be systematically tested. There are three ways to do this, which we illustrate by considering how we might answer the following question: "What is the relationship between the behavior of parents and the later delinquency of their children?"

Three Ways to Study Behavior

CROSS-SECTIONAL RESEARCH

The first method is to compare the families of very delinquent children with those of not-so-delinquent ones. Social scientists call this "cross-sectional" research because it involves examining the similarities and differences among a cross section of families studied at one point in time. It is akin to taking a snapshot. A snapshot can tell us many things—whether families with delinquent children are bigger or smaller, poorer or richer, more punitive or less punitive than families without such offspring. But it cannot tell us whether the size, the wealth, or the disciplinary practices of the families *caused* the higher rate of delinquency. In an attempt to deal with this problem, social scientists will try to hold constant every feature of the families but one to see if, after controlling for these other factors, this one factor by itself is associated with delinquency. The process is akin to sorting the snapshots, so that in one pile there are only (for example) snapshots of big, poor families, and then looking through these pictures to see if the families with harsh disciplinary practices are also the ones with more delinquent children. This sorting helps narrow down the possibilities by showing whether disciplinary practices are related to delinquency independent of family size and poverty. But this method cannot settle the question of causality. Suppose that harsh discipline occurs disproportionately among families with delinquent children. There remain three possibilities: The disciplinary practices have caused the delinquency, the existence in the family of delinquent children has caused the parents to increase the severity of their discipline, or there is some unknown third factor (perhaps a predisposition to violence) that has caused the parents to be harsh and the children to be delinquents.

LONGITUDINAL RESEARCH

The second method is to follow the development of one or more families over time. Social scientists call this "longitudinal" research. It is akin to taking, not a snapshot, but a motion picture. A motion picture helps settle the question of causality because it can tell us which factors came earlier and which later in the development of the children. If children begin misbehaving and then the parents adopt tough disciplinary practices, the latter cannot have caused the former. Even longitudinal research cannot conclusively settle the question of causality. Some unobserved changes may occur that affect the child's development in ways that lead the observer to suppose erroneously that child misbehavior caused the severe parental discipline (or vice versa). For example, the parents may have experienced some serious stress (perhaps a major illness) that caused the change in disciplinary practices but that, being unnoticed by the observer, was ignored in the causal analysis.* But though it is not perfect, the "motion-picture" method is always superior to the "snapshot" method in at least ruling out factors that could *not* have caused criminality.

Of course, getting this "motion picture" is no easy matter. One way is to start following some families from the moment they have children. Because it is forward-looking, this is called "prospective" longitudinal research. It has the great advantage that the families are picked without knowing in advance which will have delinquent children and which will not, so the results cannot be biased by the scientist's prior knowledge of the presence of delinquency. But it also has a disadvantage: Since most families will not raise high-rate offenders, a lot of the research will be wasted effort—the scientist will never see anything but trivial examples of misconduct. To solve this problem, the investigator can pick families known to have delinquent children and then ask the parents and their offspring to recall their past experiences. This is a "retrospective" longitudinal study. But as we noted earlier, such a method introduces whatever biases (and they are likely to be great) that may be caused by poor memories and deliberate misrepresentation as well as the bias caused by not knowing how normal (i.e., noncriminal) families behave. For these reasons, most scholars agree that a prospective study is superior to a retrospective one.

EXPERIMENTAL RESEARCH

The third method is to intervene deliberately in the lives of children and their families in a way that will permit the investigator to determine what effect, if any,

---

*An analogy: Doctors who have done longitudinal research on the effects of vigorous exercise on the risk of heart disease sometimes conclude that people who exercise a lot are less likely than those who are sedentary to have a heart attack. But this finding might ignore the fact that persons who exercise a lot are different from those who do not in many other ways and that these other differences may actually explain the lowered risk of heart disease.

the intervention has. This is called "experimental" research. A true experiment should randomly assign (say, by a flip of a coin) the families to either treatment or no treatment. (Those in the former group are the "experimentals," those in the latter, the "controls.") By random assignment one can ensure that the two groups differ only in the presence or absence of treatment. Hence, it is possible to demonstrate the effect, if any, of a treatment independent of all other factors.

Some investigators have tried to conduct quasi-experiments by matching (in age, sex, race, or whatever) people in a treatment program with people not in it. This can produce quite misleading results because there is always the possibility that, despite the matching, the two groups will differ in some important but unnoticed way. Indeed, given the subtlety of the factors that produce crime, it is almost certain that these differences will exist. For example, suppose a doctor treating abused children by providing them with psychotherapy wishes to find out if the treatment works. He or she creates a quasi-experiment by finding an equal number of similarly abused children who are not treated and looks at how the treated children turn out compared to the untreated ones. This is better than no experiment at all, but the results can be biased. We already know that the treated children volunteered for treatment or were referred for treatment by a social worker. Those who volunteer are likely to be quite different, psychologically and perhaps sociologically, from those who do not volunteer; similarly, children whom social workers know about and want to help may well be quite different from those the workers do not know or are not motivated to help.

A true experiment should have other features as well. There should be a long-term follow-up. Many treatments "work" for a while, simply because many people respond to anything special that is done for them, but do not have any lasting effects. There is no hard and fast rule, but in general follow-ups of less than 18 to 24 months are probably too brief. There should be several measures of the desired outcome, not just one. Most measures of crime (e.g., arrest records, conviction records, self-reported crimes) are erroneous to some degree. Using just one outcome measure may deceive the investigator into thinking that nothing has changed, when in fact something has, or into believing that there has been a change when in fact there has not. For example, a treatment may reduce the rate at which persons are arrested, but if the treatment only made the subjects more skillful in avoiding arrest, the true criminality of the subjects may not have lessened at all. And the evaluation of the experiment should be carried out by someone *other* than the therapist. A person committed, professionally and emotionally, to making some treatment work is likely to describe as successes outcomes that an impartial observer would describe as failures and to find evidence where none really exists that would justify continuing the program.

PREVIOUS STUDIES

Not many good prospective longitudinal studies or intervention experiments have been done. Of the 11 major longitudinal studies meeting certain minimal standards that have been carried out in the United States, scarcely any track closely all the likely causal factors (see Chapter 2). Most have gathered no data on the medical and physiological condition of the infant or on the mother's prenatal and perinatal experiences. Most have not attempted to assess the temperament of the child or its parents with standard psychological tests. Very few have used both arrests and self-reports as measures of criminality. Of those that have measured the child-rearing practices of the families, most have relied on occasional retrospective interviews with the parents rather than on direct observation or frequent and contemporaneous interviews. Most discuss the child's school performance, but only occasionally is there an effort to specify how early in the school years any difficulties emerged or the extent to which those difficulties are linked to learning disabilities. Almost every longitudinal study has followed only one group of children for a number of years, rather than several groups at various ages for a number of years. This means that the authors of such studies cannot know whether the development of criminal behavior in their subjects follows a pattern that will occur generally or a pattern that is unique to a group growing up in a certain period. (For example, children growing up in the 1950s, when drug abuse was relatively rare, may develop criminal careers in ways quite different from those growing up in the 1960s, when drug abuse was widespread.) Finally, the existing longitudinal studies offer little insight into the impact, if any, of efforts to change the subjects, such as special school or job-training programs.

Given the difficulty in finding opportunities to assign persons randomly to treatment or control groups and to follow up such persons over a long period, it is surprising how many criminological experiments have actually been conducted. In Chapter 3, we summarize the most important of these. In general, they test a treatment for only a short period. None shows the impact of a treatment on an entire criminal career. Only a minority of them show that the treatment had any desirable effects, and those that did show such effects tended to be prevention experiments (Schweinhart and Weikart, 1980; Feldman, Caplinger, and Wodarski, 1983). Very few successes have been reported for programs aimed at rehabilitating serious offenders, though there is some evidence that certain kinds of offenders—i.e., those that have been rather unsuccessful at crime and are young and reasonably intelligent—may benefit from some programs. Even where encouraging results can be found, they are limited to one or two relatively small experiments that have yet to be duplicated in other settings and that are vulnerable to methodological criticisms. But the occasional success story provides a glimmer of hope that is worth exploring and suggests where in the development of a criminal career may be found the best opportunity for a helpful intervention.

A New Strategy

We believe that the best way to create useful new knowledge about the prevention of crime is to mount one or more major projects that combine the strengths of longitudinal and experimental designs. In Chapter 8, we describe in some detail what such projects might be like. Though we are strongly convinced of the importance of the longitudinal-experimental method, the details we give later in this report are meant only to illustrate what the combination of these designs might be like rather than to specify a rigid, unchangeable method. The main features that we believe such a design should have are these:

MULTIPLE COHORTS

Rather than pick one group of subjects born in the same year (a "cohort") and follow them from birth to age 20 or later, we recommend picking several cohorts born in different years and following each for about six years. For example, there might be four cohorts followed from birth to age 6, 6 to 12, 12 to 18, and 18 to 24. This shortens the time until research results are obtained and enables the investigators to distinguish between the effects of aging (e.g., becoming a teenager) and the effects of an historical period (e.g., growing up in the 1990s as opposed to the 1980s). Each cohort could have about 1000 subjects.

URBAN SAMPLE

Though criminal careers can begin anywhere, crime rates are generally much higher in large cities. Moreover, choosing a cohort from a single metropolitan area permits one set of investigators located in that city to oversee all the subjects and to study the social and institutional context in which crime occurs. The metropolitan area selected should be relatively stable to minimize losses resulting from people moving out of the city. Within the area, the subjects picked should be males representative of the entire population in race and ethnicity, though it may be desirable to over-sample some groups that would have too few members in the cohort if it were picked wholly at random. The exact method of selecting subjects we leave to further inquiry. There is a case to be made for including females as well as males, but if the cohort is no larger than 1000 and half are female, the number of subjects who are likely to become high-rate offenders will be drastically reduced. (Out of 500 males, only 6 to 12%—30 to 60 persons—are likely to become serious repeat criminals; if the sample has 1000 males, then the number of repeaters rises to between 60 and 120.) Of course, the same number of repeaters (or more) could be found if the cohort of males and females totalled 2000 subjects or if the subjects were not chosen at random but by over-sampling groups known to be especially at risk for criminality. In addition to cohorts chosen from the general population, we suggest that two cohorts be selected from persons, ages 15 to 21, who have been arrested and from those, aged 18–24, who are just beginning their first prison sentences. We also suggest that, if possible, the project should be repeated in more than one metropolitan area.

MULTIPLE MEASURES OF MISCONDUCT

Data about crime should include arrest reports, self-reports, and (to the extent possible) the reports of peers, parents, and teachers. But crime and delinquency should not be the only measures of misconduct; the investigators should also gather information about disciplinary problems in the home and school, truancy, traffic violations, sexual promiscuity, alcohol and drug abuse, and employment problems.

COMPREHENSIVE INDIVIDUAL DATA

We cannot stress too much the importance of gathering information bearing on all the major causal factors that might be implicated in criminality. Every investigator will be alert to the significance of family processes, school experiences, and peer-group influences. But important as these social circumstances may be, they operate on individuals who enter this world with certain temperamental characteristics, predispositions, abilities, and weaknesses that are the product of inheritance, prenatal experiences, perinatal trauma, the events occurring during the first few months of life, or some combination of all these conditions (Wilson and Herrnstein, 1985). We do not argue that these factors "cause" crime, only that (as every parent knows) they shape the interaction between infant and caregiver and that these interactions in turn shape the personality of the child. Nor do we argue that the personality of the 1-year-old becomes the personality of the 12-year-old; people change, though there is some impressive evidence that aggression among males is one of the more stable personality factors. Failing to gather individual data, including medical and psychological factors, has the effect of ruling out these factors as contributory causes and prevents the development of programs designed to combat whatever causal power they may have.

EXPERIMENTAL TREATMENTS

A fraction of each cohort should, if possible, be randomly assigned to a treatment program, and the effect of the program should be carefully evaluated. The treatments should be selected from among those for which preliminary evidence (from existing experiments) suggests a reasonable possibility of success. Examples of possible programs follow.

The Younger Cohorts

Preschool education programs and parent training programs of the sort described in Chapter 3 might be used on a portion of the cohort to test the effect of these programs on young persons whose life histories will already be known in considerable detail. One of the difficulties in assessing the significance of such treatments (which the proposed study will overcome) is that so little is known about the behavior of the subjects before they enter the program. This means that the evaluators may underestimate the effect of the program (because the participants change in ways not evident in the standard outcome measures) or may fail to distinguish between the kinds of participants for whom the program is helpful and the kinds for whom it may be harmful.

The Older Cohorts

Older children and teenagers might be experimentally involved in programs designed to alter peer-group relationships, improve school performance, and develop resistance to alcohol and drug abuse.

The Arrested Cohorts

Persons who have been arrested might be randomly diverted from court or exposed to some degree of punishment appropriate to their offense, or randomly assigned to juvenile or adult court.

Imprisoned Cohorts

The effect on imprisoned persons of different release patterns (early release on parole, release on work furlough) or different conditions of release (with or without financial assistance or job placement) has been tested already, but not with the detailed information about the inmates' life histories that this project envisions. With this rich body of information, it should be possible to disentangle positive, negative, and neutral influences so that we would know for what kinds of inmates particular programs have desirable or undesirable effects.

Organizing for Research

No project of the size and complexity we are proposing has ever been attempted in criminological or criminal justice research. Because it is unprecedented, it is especially risky. But it is not unacceptably risky. Even if many of the experiments cannot be carried out owing to organizational, financial, or legal problems, we will still have gathered an extraordinarily valuable body of information about the natural history of criminal and noncriminal careers. Moreover, analogous projects have been undertaken in other fields. It is not uncommon, for example, for large cohorts of subjects to be carefully followed for many years in medical research and for special treatments (e.g., reducing blood cholesterol levels) to be given to some members of the cohort.

We have relatively little to say about the organizational structure or structures within which this project should be undertaken. The Justice Program Study Group commissioned a number of papers from scholars around the United States who proposed various methods for designing and executing longitudinal and experimental research and held a conference at which these papers were discussed. It is clear that further work needs to be done before the final design and structure can be settled upon. We are not certain whether one entity (for example, a university-based research group) should design and manage the research as a single project or whether several allied research groups should collaborate in designing the research with data gathering left to a specialized organization. We are not certain of the right mix of governmental and private funds with which to support this venture. (We estimate that it may cost $1 million per year for several years, but the cost could be higher if the size of the cohorts or the number of experiments was increased.)

Moreover, we do not wish to undercut other research strategies. A great deal has been learned using cross-sectional methods. By taking these snapshots and analyzing their contents, we have learned about the role of alcohol and heroin in certain kinds of crime, the extent to which victims sometimes precipitate attacks on themselves, the degree to which juvenile crime occurs in groups, the association between school failure and delinquency, and the psychological differences among types of offenders. Through retrospective longitudinal studies, we have learned about the kinds of persons who become high-rate as opposed to low-rate offenders and the association between criminality and intelligence, family discord, and unemployment. Indeed, it is only possible to grasp the potential benefits of a prospective longitudinal study that includes experimental interventions by drawing on what we already have learned from different research methods.

Progress in medicine came from research and experimentation. Some of that research was catch-as-catch-can—trying a new drug or treatment to see if it helped arrest the course of a serious ailment. In time, methods for testing more accurately the effects of new drugs were developed, so that today checking the efficacy and safety of new products has become routine. But it gradually became clear to physicians that, if serious diseases were to be prevented rather than simply treated, scientists would have to study sick people to see how they got that way (retrospective longitudinal research) and healthy people to see what caused some to become ill (prospective longitudinal research). Groups of persons—cohorts—were followed for years to learn about the effects on health of heavy smoking, high levels of cholesterol, and exposure to various environmental hazards. The lesson of these complex, long-term projects was the discovery that society may be underinvesting in preventing illness and overinvesting in treating illness, given the relative gains to be had from prevention and treatment.

Research today on how best to deal with crime is no further along than was research in the 19th century on how best to deal with illness. We have learned some clues on how to treat some problems and we have a pretty good idea about what the "very sick patient" (i.e., the high-rate offender) looks like and what his circumstances have been. But we have only the most rudimentary ideas about the developmental sequence of criminality and thus we have only a few tantalizing clues as to where in that sequence we might intervene with good effect.

It may be that there is no way we can intervene on any large scale. The causes of crime may be buried so deeply in the human psyche, intimate family processes, and profound cultural norms that we cannot learn how to make meaningful changes or, if we do learn, we would find the necessary methods to be abhorrent. We may have to content ourselves with dealing with symptoms rather than causes and doing so on the basis of the rather crude instruments now at our disposal, such as police officers, target hardening, prisons, fines, and drug treatment programs.

We do not know whether to be optimistic or pessimistic. We do know that we have not tried very hard to find out. There have been hundreds of important studies of the effects of smoking on health; there have been but a handful on what many people would regard as a far graver public-health problem—criminality. We believe we can do better, and that we should. We are aware that many readers would prefer to reject our recommendations in favor of quick action to implement plausible schemes that seem to have immediate payoffs. We do not wish to dissuade them from doing whatever seems constructive in the short run. But we do urge them to set aside some time, effort, and money to prepare better for the long term. We are also aware that some readers, noting that crime rates have been flat or declining for the last few years, will conclude that the crisis is over and that major new studies of criminal careers are unnecessary. We remind them that our society was caught completely unprepared for the extraordinary increase in crime during the 1960s and 1970s, that many people may have suffered needlessly as a result, that crime rates will go up again in the future, and that we are not much better prepared for the next crime wave than we were for the last.

Finally, we wish to stress that, though our principal charge has been to make recommendations regarding crime, our strategy, if it is of any value at all, will have benefits that go well beyond any crime-reduction potential. People who frequently commit crimes are not normal in all other aspects of their lives. For the high-rate offender, crime is usually but one manifestation of a life that is generally disorderly and pathological. The high-rate offender tends also to be the failing student, the drunken driver, the unreliable employee, and the abusive or neglectful parent. An inquiry into the causes of criminality is at the same time an inquiry into the causes of general defects in character and behavior; lessons learned about how to prevent crime will almost surely be lessons learned about how to produce better citizens. Scholars in many fields in addition to criminology will find the data of a major longitudinal–experimental study of great value in understanding how to help people who constitute not just a large fraction of the workload of practitioners in criminal justice, but also of those in education, social work, mental health, and manpower development. We hope that agencies interested in such matters will lend their support to this venture. If it succeeds for one, it is likely to succeed for all.

The Plan of the Book

The remainder of this book spells out these conclusions and recommendations in greater detail. Chapters 2 and 3 review what we have learned from the relatively few longitudinal and experimental studies that have been carried out. The reader will note that, in general, longitudinal studies have not included experimental interventions and experimental studies have not involved a long-term follow-up. Chapters 4 through 7 discuss some key policy issues that require further research if we are to do a better job in preventing or treating crime and delinquency. Chapter 4 reviews the role of families and schools in delinquency, Chapter 5 discusses the controversy over labeling, Chapter 6 analyzes proposals for redirecting the juvenile court, and Chapter 7 considers the effects, insofar as they are known, of imprisonment.

There are many other issues that could have been added to this list, but the conclusions would have been essentially the same: If policymakers are to take a sensible position on how best to prevent delinquency and handle offenders, they must know more than is now known. In Chapter 8 we outline the kinds of longitudinal–experimental studies that are needed to advance our knowledge and resolve some of the dilemmas facing policymakers.

2
What Have We Learned From Major Longitudinal Surveys?

Introduction

Uses and Advantages of Longitudinal Surveys

Longitudinal surveys involve *repeated* measures of the same people or of samples from the same population or of other units (such as areas). They can be compared with cross-sectional surveys, in which information is collected at one time only. The major advantage of longitudinal surveys lies in their ability to provide detailed information about the natural history and course of development of a phenomenon. In discussions about crime, the major phenomenon of interest is the criminal career.

Most of the key questions about the explanation, prevention, and treatment of crime are essentially questions about criminal careers. Why do people start committing crimes? Why do they continue to commit crimes? Why does the frequency or seriousness of their crimes increase? Why do people stop committing crimes? Why do people switch from one kind of crime to another? Why does the prevalence of crime peak in the teenage years? How can the typical course of criminal careers be changed? At what point is it best to intervene? How can people be deterred or reformed? How many crimes are prevented by imprisoning people for a certain period? For all these questions, and others that could be posed, we need detailed knowledge about the time course of criminal careers.

Longitudinal research can show when criminal careers begin, when they end, and how long they last. It can also show the prevalence and incidence of offending, the cumulative prevalence rate, and the seriousness and diversity of offending, at different ages or stages of a criminal career.

It can also demonstrate continuities and discontinuities in criminal careers, the extent to which offenders tend to specialize in types of offenses during their careers, and the extent to which the most frequent or serious offenders at one age tend to be the most frequent and serious offenders at another. It can also show the relation between earlier and later events, and the extent to which different aspects of criminal careers can be predicted. Another advantage of longitudinal research is that it can provide information about the time ordering of different events, which can be useful in drawing conclusions about cause and effect. In addition, it can show the effects of different events on the course of development of criminal careers and the extent to which different aspects of them are transmitted from one generation to the next. (These topics are discussed in more detail in the section "What Have We Learned?"; see also Farrington, 1979c).

Cross-sectional research cannot generate adequate information about criminal careers. For example, cross-sectional data can show the prevalence and incidence of offending at different ages but cannot show how offending at one age is linked to offending at another. The prevalence of many property crimes seems to peak about age 17, while the corresponding peak for violent crimes is around age 24 (Cline, 1980). Longitudinal research, unlike cross-sectional studies, can show whether the property offenders diversify into violence as they get older or whether the property offenders desist and a new group of violent offenders emerges.

To take another example, cross-sectional research shows that drug use declines dramatically after age 40. However, this decline may reflect period effects rather than aging. There was a massive increase in drug use during the late 1960s. It could be argued that persons now over 40 have low rates of drug use because they were not exposed to such widespread drug influences during their formative (teenage) years, rather than because drug use declines precipitously with age. It seems unlikely that those who were teenagers in the late 1960s will have similarly low rates when they are over 40, but only longitudinal surveys, preferably following up cohorts born in different years, can distinguish between period and aging effects.

A major problem in using the cross-sectional method to study changes over time is that any differences between groups may not be connected with time. For example, a group of persons now aged 20 and living in an area may differ in many ways other than age from a group now aged 30 and living in the same area, because of immigration, emigration, and deaths. In a different context (studying the effects of imprisonment), a group of persons who have now served one year in prison may differ in many ways other than time served from a group who have now served five years in prison. Longitudinal research can avoid or control for such selection effects by following up the same people over time. Essentially, each person acts as his or her own control. Therefore, in longitudinal research, differences between those aged 20 and those aged 30 do not reflect preexisting differences between different groups but reflect changes over time.

There are some advantages of cross-sectional studies. In particular, there is the practical advantage that they can usually be carried out more easily, quickly, and cheaply than longitudinal ones. Another advantage is that cross-sectional studies are not susceptible to testing effects, when the experience of being interviewed changes people and may affect their responses in the next interview. It is desirable to estimate the magnitude of testing effects in a longitudinal survey by testing only subsamples or by comparing a subsample seen frequently with one seen rarely. When this has been done (Douglas, 1970; Bachman, O'Malley, and Johnston, 1978), observed testing effects have been small.

There are also advantages in combining cross-sectional and longitudinal research. For example, in following up one cohort, it is often difficult to know if changes over time reflect changes with age or changes over the historical period. These two factors could be disentangled by following up several different cohorts who reach different ages in the same year (and vice versa). However, a more economical approach might be to combine a longitudinal survey with two cross-sectional surveys, one at the start of the period and one at the end. In following up a cohort from age 10 in 1980 to age 20 in 1990, cross-sectional surveys could be done with persons aged 10 to 20 in 1980 and again with persons aged 10 to 20 in 1990.

In the context of a discussion about the relation between age and crime, Hirschi and Gottfredson (1983) argued that longitudinal studies were unnecessary. Since this view clearly conflicts with our own, we feel it is incumbent upon us to consider their arguments. Their basic points are that the relation between age and crime is invariant and that the causes of crime at one age are the same as those at any other age. Hence, cross-sectional research is sufficient to specify both the time course of criminal careers and the causes of crime at different ages.

We do not agree with either of these arguments. First of all, the relation between age and crime is not invariant. Indeed, the relation as obtained by cross-sectional data is often different from that obtained longitudinally (Farrington, 1979c, 1986a). Furthermore, the age–crime relationship is different for different kinds of offenses (Cline, 1980). Second, there are different relationships with offending at different ages. For example, in the London longitudinal survey (discussed later), Farrington (1986c) reported that if a child, up to age 10, had parents who had been convicted, this was one of the best predictors of that child offending at ages 14 through 16 and 17 through 20, but it did not predict offending at ages 10 through 13. West (1982) reported that if a delinquent married between ages 18 and 21, marriage had no effect on offending between these ages, while marriage between 21 and 24 (to a noncriminal woman) led to a decrease in offending between these ages. It is implausible to propose that a variable such as marriage should have the same effect on offending at all ages. Even if this were true cross-sectionally (between subjects), longitudinal relationships (within subjects) are far more important in drawing conclusions about causes, prevention, and treatment. Consequently, we do not agree with Hirschi and Gottfredson's argument that longitudinal studies are unnecessary.

Most research on crime and delinquency has been and is cross-sectional in design. Nevertheless, most of our firm knowledge about criminal careers derives from longitudinal studies. This chapter will review the major longitudinal surveys that have been carried out and the major advances in our knowledge that have resulted up to the present time, giving some attention to the practical and policy implications.

Desirable Features of Longitudinal Surveys

Longitudinal surveys can be prospective or retrospective. Studies that are prospective, in collecting data contemporaneously with or soon after the events of interest (and usually before key outcomes such as adult criminal behavior), are especially useful. In prospective studies, the data collection can be designed in advance to test hypothesis specified by the researcher. Also, it cannot be biased by a knowledge of later outcomes.

In retrospective longitudinal research, people are often asked to remember events that happened several years before. For example, in the Rand research of Petersilia, Greenwood, and Lavin (1978), adult prisoners were asked about offenses they had committed during their juvenile, young adult, and adult years. The memories of people who are trying to provide information about past events may be not only faulty but also affected by retrospective bias (see Chess and Thomas, 1984, p. 6). For example, consider a mother of a 15-year-old convicted male who is attempting to answer questions about how she brought him up. The methods of child rearing she used before the conviction are likely to be of most relevance to the investigator who is interested in explaining delinquency because methods used afterward may have been affected by it. However, the problem is that the mother's memory of the child-rearing methods used beforehand may be affected by the conviction. Many people search for explanations for delinquency, and the mother may feel that her child-rearing methods must have been unsatisfactory because her son became a convicted delinquent.

Just as prospective surveys have more scope for testing hypotheses than retrospective ones, so surveys in which records are supplemented by data from interviews have more scope than those based on records alone. Most longitudinal surveys of crime and delinquency have been based entirely on official criminal records. Many of these have greatly increased our knowledge. For example, the two most significant contributors to our knowledge about criminal careers have been Blumstein (see Blumstein, Cohen, and Hsieh, 1982) and Wolfgang (see Wolfgang, Figlio, and Sellin, 1972), both using surveys of this kind. Similarly, our knowledge about careers of criminal violence has been advanced considerably by the Ohio Dangerous Offenders project, again entirely based on official records (Hamparian, Schuster, Dinitz, and Conrad, 1978; Van Dine, Conrad, and Dinitz, 1979; Miller, Dinitz, and Conrad, 1982).

There are many problems with research based only on records. First of all, the researcher is limited by the information available in the records. The researcher is not free to specify the questions in advance and to make sure, by appropriate research design, that that information necessary to answer them is collected. Second, concentration on criminal records may blind researchers to the continuity that exists between crime and other kinds of socially disapproved behavior. One of the most important contributions of Robins' (1966, 1978) longitudinal surveys was to demonstrate the versatility of antisocial behavior as well as its continuity from childhood to adulthood. In her 30-year follow-up of children referred to a child guidance clinic in St. Louis, she found that the children stole, were truants, ran away from home, were aggressive, enuretic, disciplinary problems in school, pathological liars, and so on. As adults, they tended to be arrested, divorced, placed in mental hospitals, sexually promiscuous, vagrants, bad debtors, poor workers, and so on. Research based only on criminal records may lose sight of the fact that criminal behavior may be only one element of a much larger social problem.

Another difficulty with records collected by the police and other criminal justice agencies is that they form a biased and underrepresentative sample of all delinquent or criminal acts committed. Also, records are kept for the benefit of agency personnel rather than researchers; they are often kept inefficiently or unsystematically, and legal categories may distort the real behavior that occurred. There are many reasons why criminal acts fail to appear in an official record; failure to define the act as criminal, failure to report the act to the police, failure to record the act by the police, and failure to apprehend any offender. The major problem is that official records of crime reflect the behavior of both offenders and official agencies, and it is difficult to disentangle them.

If the subjects of the survey are interviewed, it is possible to ask them about criminal acts they have committed and, hence, collect self-reports of acts that have not necessarily come to the notice of the police. It is important to study undetected as well as detected offenses in order to obtain a complete picture. Self-report measures of offending are not free from problems, of course. Some members of the sample will not be available for interview, and there is some evidence that the worst offenders tend to be the most elusive respondents (West and Farrington, 1973). Those who are interviewed might conceal, exaggerate, or forget their offenses. Many self-report questionnaires are overweighted with relatively trivial items that, although technically crimes, would rarely lead to official processing. The validity of self-reports has usually been investigated by comparing them with official records (e.g., Farrington, 1973; Hindelang, Hirschi, and Weis, 1981), and it has been found that crimes that have been recorded are usually also reported by the subjects. As in other cases, it is desirable to have at least two measures of the same theoretical construct, inevitably subject to different biases. If results obtained with official records hold up with self-reports, this would increase our confidence in conclusions drawn about criminal behavior (rather than the conclusions reflecting police selection or self-report bias).

Very few longitudinal surveys have interviewed the subjects repeatedly. In a number of cases, a (usually retrospective) search of records has been combined with one interview, and this has provided more information than the records alone. For example, later work on the Wolfgang survey of Philadelphia boys born in 1945 (Wolfgang, 1980; Thornberry and Farnworth, 1982) included an interview at age 26, and Shannon (1981) interviewed some of the first two of his Racine, Wisconsin, cohorts at ages 34 and 27, respectively. The two long-term surveys by Robins (Robins, 1966; Robins, West, and Herjanic, 1975) also included one interview when the subjects were aged at least 30. These famous surveys will be discussed in more detail later.

As an example of a longitudinal survey in which one interview was followed by a search of records, Feldhusen and his collaborators (Feldhusen, Thurston, and Benning, 1973; Feldhusen, Aversano, and Thurston, 1976) were interested in predicting delinquency. All teachers in Eau Claire County, Wisconsin, were asked to identify third, sixth, and ninth grade children who were persistently aggressive or disruptive and other children who were consistently well behaved. Nearly 200 of each kind were then interviewed and tested in their schools and subsequently followed up in records for 8 years. About half of the aggressive children acquired a police record for nontraffic offenses, and delinquency was predicted by such factors as sex, grade level, IQ, and degree of behavior problems.

In several surveys, the subjects have been followed up using telephone interviews or mail questionnaires rather than by means of face-to-face personal interviews. Both mail and telephone were used by Havighurst, Bowman, Liddle, Matthews, and Pierce (1962). They initially contacted nearly 500 children in a midwestern city at ages 11 through 14 during 1951–54, obtaining teacher and peer ratings, and followed them up to 1960 by mail and by telephone. They found that delinquency was predicted by such factors as low social class, school failure, and rated aggression in the sixth grade.

Other mail follow-ups were completed by Polk et al. (1981) and Bachman et al. (1978). Both of these were large-scale studies of the development of delinquent or criminal careers in representative samples. Polk et al. tracked over 1,200 high school boys from Marion County, Oregon, who completed a questionnaire in 1964, attempting to interview a subsample in 1968 and following up to 1979 using mail questionnaires. They also collected official records of juvenile and adult offending. Bachman et al. in the Youth in Transition study tracked a nationally representative sample of over 2,200 boys aged about 15 in 1966. These boys were interviewed in 1966 and 1968, given group-administered questionnaires in 1969 and 1970, and followed up in 1974 by means of mail questionnaires. The researchers measured offending entirely by self-report.

It seems likely that telephone interviews and mail questionnaires, while relatively easy to carry out, might be less reliable and valid than personal face-to-face interviews. In face-to-face interviews, it should be possible to collect more extensive and more sensitive information, and it might be harder for the subject to present a false picture (e.g., about home conditions, which might be obvious during home interviews). Therefore, face-to-face interviews are to be preferred.

Surprisingly few longitudinal surveys of crime and delinquency involving two or more interviews with the subjects have been carried out in the United States. Even when such studies have been conducted, the results have sometimes been presented in such a way that it is impossible to draw conclusions about criminal behavior, and this is especially true of predominantly psychiatric investigations. For example, in studying long-term relationships between physique and criminal behavior, Hartl, Monnelly, and Elderkin (1982) followed up the 200 Boston men originally seen in 1939 by Sheldon, Hartl, and McDermott (1949). These men were interviewed in 1958 and 1963 and contacted by letter (and in some cases by telephone) four more times up to 1979. Unfortunately, the results are presented as complete case histories and psychiatric categories, providing no useful information about the topics reviewed in the section "What We Have Learned?"

It has been argued so far that the most valuable longitudinal surveys are those that are prospective and include face-to-face interviews as well as records. Other desirable features of a longitudinal survey are that it should cover a reasonable time period (at least five years) and include a reasonably large sample (in the hundreds at least). The longer the survey, the better the complete, natural history of a phenomenon can be studied, as opposed to what can be gleaned from a "snapshot," which pays little attention to the events leading up to or following the phenomenon. Also, surveys including less than 100 subjects have a rather limited ability to study crime and delinquency because, apart from the obvious problem of generalization to a population, they will often include too few of the most criminal persons in the community. This was true, for example, of the study by Peck and Havighurst (1960). In a midwestern community, they followed up 34 children from age 10 to age 18, interviewing the children, their parents, and their friends every year.

There are other features of longitudinal surveys that are desirable but rarely found. In particular, it would be valuable to have data collected at intervals not greater than one year. To some extent, the optimal interval depends on the speed of developmental change, which needs to be studied at different ages for different phenomena.

Frequent data collection is also necessary in establishing the relative timing or ordering of events. For example, Farrington could demonstrate (1977) that convictions were followed by an increase in self-reported delinquency and could show (1978) that newly emerging parental disharmony at age 14 preceded newly emerging aggressive behavior at ages 16 to 18. Information about time order is essential in trying to establish causal order in nonexperimental research, although (as pointed out in Chapter 3) causal relationships can be demonstrated most effectively in longitudinal research combined with experimentation. Another advantage of repeated data collection is its ability to establish reliability and validity. When subjects are being seen repeatedly, it is hard for them to present a false picture of themselves to researchers without being detected.

Another desirable feature of a longitudinal survey is that data should be collected from a variety of different sources—official records, interviews with the subjects, and interviews with other informants such as parents, peers, and teachers. This helps to establish how consistent behavior is in different settings (see Loeber and Dishion, 1984). It also helps to determine the validity of measures and to disentangle real findings from ones produced artifactually by common response biases (as pointed out above). For example, if self-reports of offending were related to self-reports of attachment to parents and self-reports of school success, it could always be argued that the relationships were produced artifactually by common self-report biases. In other words, some people were willing to tell researchers about socially disapproved topics and others were not. On the other hand, if self-reports of offending were related to parent reports of attachment and teacher reports of school success, it would be more plausible to conclude that offending, attachment, and school success are related. Also, there may be advantages in deriving composite variables by combining measures from different sources or at different ages. Such variables may contain less bias or error than the constituent measures because errors may tend to be in opposite directions and hence may cancel out to some extent in the combined variable.

Very few longitudinal surveys possess the desirable features outlined in this section. The most important ones will be described next.

Major Prospective Longitudinal Surveys

It seems that there are only 11 American longitudinal surveys that fulfill all the following criteria: (a) prospective, (b) two or more interviews with the subjects, (c) the first and last interview separated by at least five years, (d) a sample in the hundreds at least, and (e) a body of information about criminal or delinquent behavior. It is these kinds of major longitudinal surveys that are the focus of this chapter. In this report, we are particularly concerned with advancing knowledge about the most frequent and serious offenders and offenses and especially about violent crimes, predatory crimes such as robbery, and property offenses such as burglary. Hence, we are most interested in longitudinal surveys that provide information about the high-rate offender.

Three of these were carried out by those pioneers of follow-up research, the Gluecks. The first survey (Glueck and Glueck, 1930, 1937, 1943) followed up about 500 men (average age 25) whose sentences in a Massachusetts reformatory expired during 1921–22 and interviewed them or their relatives 5, 10, and 15 years later. The second (Glueck and Glueck, 1934, 1940) followed up 1,000 juvenile delinquents (average age 14) examined by the Judge Baker Clinic in Boston during 1917–22 and interviewed them or their relatives 5 or 15 years later. The third survey (Glueck and Glueck, 1950, 1968) followed up 500 delinquents in Massachusetts correctional schools during 1939–44 and 500 matched nondelinquents. These boys were contacted initially at an average age of 14, and later at average ages of 25 and 31.

The Gluecks' surveys were important for a number of reasons. First, they showed the feasibility of long-term follow-ups. Usually, nearly half of the sample could be interviewed personally; in another one-third of cases, close relatives could be seen. Second, they provided information about the long-term careers of detected offenders, not only about crimes committed at different ages but also about other aspects of life such as work history and marital adjustment. The recidivism rates were often depressingly high; for example, of the 1,000 juvenile delinquents followed up for the first five years, 77 did not have reliable information, 18 had no opportunity to commit offenses, and 798 of the remaining 905 (88%) were officially recorded for further offenses (Glueck and Glueck, 1934).

The Gluecks also studied in some detail the factors that predicted recidivism, developing prediction tables based on between five and seven factors. For example, taking again the 1,000 juvenile delinquents followed up for five years, the best predictors of recidivism were paternal discipline, maternal discipline, school retardation, school misconduct, and the age of the first known behavior disorder. The Gluecks' methods of selecting and combining factors into a prediction table can be criticized (see, e.g., Farrington and Tarling, 1985), but their careful documentation of variables that predicted offending was clearly an important step forward.

Two of the 11 surveys were carried out by Hathaway and Monachesi (1957, 1963; see also Wirt and Briggs, 1959; Hathaway, Monachesi, and Young, 1960; Hathaway, Reynolds, and Monachesi, 1969). Both initially involved boys and girls, but only the boys were included in the long-term delinquency follow-ups. The first survey involved nearly 2,000 boys (average age 15) tested in Minneapolis during 1947–48. Selected samples were contacted 4 and 8 years later. The second involved 5,700 boys (average age 15) tested in Minnesota schools during 1953–54, contacting selected samples at ages 19 and 28.

The main aim of these surveys was to investigate to what extent delinquency could be predicted by the Minnesota Multiphasic Personality Inventory (MMPI). Their results showed that the development of delinquency in previously nondelinquent boys could be predicted to some extent, and Hathaway and Monachesi (1957) even presented a 33-item MMPI scale designed to predict delinquency. Most of the items on the scale referred to the boy's own misbehavior (e.g., "During one period while I was a youngster, I engaged in petty thievery"—True) or to his liking for risky activities (e.g., "I have never done anything dangerous for the thrill of it"—False).

The longest lasting American longitudinal survey of crime and delinquency is the Cambridge–Somerville Youth Study begun by Powers and Witmer (1951) and continued by McCord, McCord, and Zola (1959) and McCord (1978, 1979). Initially, during 1937–39 in Massachusetts, 650 boys (average age 10) were nominated by schools (as difficult or average) and enrolled in the study. Half, chosen at random, were given rather heterogeneous social work treatment (or "friendly visiting" according to Vosburgh and Alexander, 1980) for an average of five years. On the basis of the records made by the visiting counselors during this period, the boys' parents were rated on such factors as attitudes (cruel, passive, or neglecting), discipline (lax or erratic), and quarrelsomeness. Thirty years after the end of the treatment, McCord attempted to follow up 506 who had at least four years of treatment, initially by mail questionnaires and later by interview.

The social work treatment did not have the desired effect, as will be discussed in more detail in the chapter on experimental research (Chapter 3). The results of the longitudinal analyses are also interesting. For example, McCord (1979) reported that maternal supervision predicted convictions for property offenses and violence, while maternal affection and paternal deviance (alcoholism or convictions) predicted property offenses only, and parental conflict and parental aggression predicted violence only. In another interesting analysis, McCord (1982) showed that broken homes (caused by loss of the biological father) with affectionate mothers were not more likely to produce convicted children than united homes without conflict. United homes with conflict and broken homes without affectionate mothers were both more criminogenic.

Another long-lasting survey was carried out by Lefkowitz, Eron, Walder, and Huesmann (1977). Their research is interesting because of its combination of interview and record data with peer ratings and parent reports. They initially interviewed 875 children aged 8–9 during 1959–60 in New York State and followed them up at ages 18–19 and 30 (Eron, 1982). Unlike the earlier surveys by the Gluecks and by Hathaway and Monachesi, they carried out multivariate analyses to investigate the extent to which factors predicted aggression independently of other factors. One of their major results was that the best predictor of peer-rated aggression for males at age 18–19 was a preference for watching violent television programs at age 8–9. However, this result did not hold for females. Also, they found surprising consistency in aggressiveness from age 8 to age 30 for both sexes.

Another project that is interesting because of its multiple cohort design was carried out by Langner, Gersten, and Eisenberg (1977) in New York City. They surveyed two samples of about 1,000 children initially aged 6–18, one randomly selected and the other derived from households receiving Aid to Dependent Children. The mothers and subsamples of the children were interviewed during 1967–68 and again about five years later. The best predictors of delinquency in the children were punitive parents and rejecting mothers.

A follow-up study of nearly 700 children was carried out in Hawaii by Werner and Smith (1982). The children were tracked from birth in 1955 to age 18. The mothers were interviewed before and just after the children were born, and the subjects themselves were interviewed at age 10 and (subsamples) at age 18. Werner and Smith found that children who developed delinquency or mental health problems tended to have experienced parental discord, a mother who had mental health problems, a father who lost his job, and a mother who became pregnant again within two years of the child's birth. They also studied why some children with these risk factors nevertheless led successful, law-abiding lives and found that the resilient boys (in comparison with others) tended to be first born, to be from smaller families characterized by low discord, and to display high infant intelligence at age 2.

The full results of another interesting project have not yet been published; a Chicago study carried out by Kellam, Branch, Brown, and Russell (1981) during which they interviewed parents and children. Their sample consisted of more than 1,200 families with first-grade children in 1966 and 1967. The children were interviewed at about ages 6, 8, and 16, and the final interview included a self-reported delinquency questionnaire.

The most recent American longitudinal survey of the type described above is one of the most influential criminological studies of the present time. Elliott and Huizinga (1983) and Ageton (1983) have followed up 1,725 adolescents (out of a nationally representative target sample of 2,360) aged 11–17 in 1976, interviewing them every year until 1981. A sixth round of interviews was completed in 1984. The latest interviews make this the first American longitudinal survey of crime and delinquency involving a good-sized sample and more than three interviews spanning at least five years. An additional advantage of the project is that both official records and self-reports of the offending have been collected. The survey does not include information from any source other than official records and the subjects themselves, except for a short questionnaire completed by parents at the time of the first interview. The results of this survey will be discussed in detail in the section "What Have We Learned?"

Moving outside the United States, there has been a substantial amount of longitudinal research on crime and delinquency in Great Britain and in the Scandinavian countries. In Great Britain, the pioneering study was the National Survey of Health and Development, directed initially by Douglas and later by Wadsworth (see Douglas, Ross, and Simpson, 1968; Wadsworth, 1979). This was a follow-up of more than 5,300 children selected from all legitimate single births in England, Scotland, and Wales in one week of March 1946. Data was collected at one- or two-year intervals at least up to age 21, usually by questionnaires filled in by health visitors or teachers. The criminal records of the children were studied up to the twenty-first birthday, and it emerged that large family size and separations due to reasons other than death or hospitalization were important predictors of delinquency.

A more restricted area study was carried out by Miller, Court, Knox, and Brandon (1974). A representative sample of more than 1,100 children born in Newcastle in 1947 was followed from birth to age 15. As in the National Survey, the children and their families were contacted at regular intervals (usually every year) by health visitors, and information was also obtained from teachers. The final attempt to contact the sample was made at age 22, although criminal records have now been collected up to ages 32 and 33. As observed in many other studies, those who became delinquents tended to have suffered many disadvantages, ranging from low social class, unemployed fathers, and large families to low IQ and low heights and weights.

A third British longitudinal survey was directed by West and Farrington (1973, 1977). They followed up more than 400 London boys from age 8 in 1961 and 1962 to age 25. The boys themselves were interviewed seven times, and an eighth interview (at ages 31 and 32) began toward the end of 1984. The boys' parents were also interviewed yearly as long as the boys were in school, and their teachers and peers also filled in questionnaires at intervals. Criminal records were obtained not only for the boys but also for their fathers, mothers, brothers, sisters, and wives. The regularly collected self-reports of offending were compared with the official records. This criminological survey is unique in covering more than 20 years, in the number of personal interviews with hundreds of subjects, and in the variety of sources of data. It will be discussed in more detail in the section "What Have We Learned?"

The most interesting Scandinavian longitudinal surveys of crime and delinquency are probably the two versions of *Project Metropolitan* carried out in Copenhagen and Stockholm (see Janson, 1981; Hogh and Wolf, 1981). This project, inspired by the British National Survey, was originally intended to be completed in all four Scandinavian countries. In Copenhagan, all (12,000) boys born in 1953 were tested in school in 1965 and 1966, and a subsample of their mothers was interviewed in 1968. In Stockholm, all (15,000) children born in 1953 were tested in school in 1966, and a subsample of their mothers was interviewed in 1968. Both groups were followed up in police records, in Stockholm up to 1978 and in Copenhagen up to 1976 (according to the most recent published information).

Another important Scandinavian criminological survey was completed by Magnusson, Duner, and Zetterblom (1975). Three cohorts of about 1,000 children born in Orebro, Sweden (a town of about 100,000 inhabitants), in 1950, 1952, and 1955 were followed up from 1965 to 1971. The researchers hope to track these children further into adult life using criminal and other records (see Magnusson and Duner, 1981). This study is especially worthy of note because of the variety of sources of data. Information from the subjects was supplemented by peer, parent, and teacher ratings, records, and a number of interesting biological measures. One of the most important results so far shows the ability of the teachers' ratings of aggression to predict later delinquency.

As will be seen from the foregoing discussion, most existing longitudinal surveys have been concerned with predicting delinquency, usually as a prelude to explaining it. However, there are great problems in this essentially nonexperimental research method in moving from prediction to explanation. As mentioned in Chapter 1, almost everything that is measured tends to predict delinquency. The emphasis in the section "What Have We Learned?" will be on establishing basic facts about criminal careers.

Studies Based On Larger Units

In all the projects mentioned above, individuals were followed up. In some cases, information was also collected from other family members, but the focus of interest was on individuals rather than families. Similarly, data was sometimes obtained from schools or peer groups about the individuals of interest.

Longitudinal research on crime and delinquency could involve the tracking of larger units than individuals, such as families, schools, peer groups (e.g., gangs), communities, areas, or penal institutions. This kind of project would be especially desirable if the criminal behavior of the larger unit was not merely the sum of the criminal behavior of the individuals in it. To take an obvious example, if delinquent acts are committed by groups rather than by lone individuals, the total number of acts committed may be overestimated if each individual is counted separately. This depends to some extent on the answer to the question: What is a crime? If three people acting together break into a house, should that be counted as one burglary or three? A victim survey would disclose only one burglary, while a self-reported offending survey (unless it contained specific questions about group size and took account of this) would disclose three. The usual rule in official criminal statistics is that one victim equals one crime, but this seems unrealistic in some cases. For example, if three men acting together rape one woman, this seems to be three acts of rape rather than one.

A great deal of delinquency is committed in groups (Zimring, 1981). However, it is not clear whether peers tend to encourage or facilitate offending or whether the high prevalence of group offending merely reflects the fact that, when adolescents go out, they tend to go out in groups. Whatever the explanation, the group nature of offending suggests that attempts should be made to link up individual criminal careers and to follow up groups. Also, it is noticeable that offending tends to be concentrated in families. West and Farrington (1977) found that 4.6% of their families accounted for 48% of all the convictions of nuclear family members (fathers, mothers, sons, and daughters). This suggests that it might be worthwhile to link up and follow up the careers of all members of a nuclear family.

As with the study of individuals, longitudinal research on larger units should be concerned with what medical researchers call epidemiology: the differential distribution of crime over the units or aspects of the units, and the correlation between this distribution and environmental or individual factors. One of the most famous, classic uses of epidemiology in uncovering the causes of infectious disease was based on larger units than individuals. In 19th century London, Snow noticed that the distribution of cases of cholera seemed to follow the pattern of water supply. Various checks indicated that this association was unlikely to be due to any other factors and Snow came to the conclusion that the water from particular pumps was probably causing the cholera. He then carried out an experiment that confirmed this. The Broad Street pump was closed, and this had the predicted effect of reducing cases of cholera (see Rutter, 1981).

Criminological research based on areas is often referred to as ecological research, following the pioneering work of Shaw and McKay (1969) in Chicago and five other cities. Shaw and McKay found that the distribution of juvenile delinquents' residences followed patterns of physical structure and social organization in cities. Generally, juvenile delinquents were concentrated in areas of physical deterioration and neighborhood disorganization. A large proportion of offenders came from a small proportion of areas in Chicago. Furthermore, the distribution of delinquency was surprisingly consistent over time. For juvenile court appearances, for example, the distribution during 1900–06 correlated .61 with the distribution during 1927–33.

Shaw and McKay concluded that variations in delinquency reflected variations in the social values and norms to which children were exposed, which tended to be consistent over time in any given area. They argued that because delinquency was caused by social disorganization, it could be prevented by community organization. This idea led to the Chicago Area Project, which aimed to coordinate community resources to increase the educational, recreational, and occupational opportunities for young people. The success of this in reducing delinquency has never been rigorously demonstrated (Schlossman and Sedlak, 1983).

Shaw and McKay's theories have been extremely influential in the history of criminology. Many other ecological studies have been carried out (for a review, see Baldwin, 1979) but hardly any have had a longitudinal design. One exception is the study by Schmid (1960) in Seattle. He reported high correlations between the distribution of the locations of offenses during 1939–41 and the distribution during 1949–51.

The most important recent longitudinal study of areas was carried out in Chicago by Bursik and Webb (1982). Pointing out that most of Shaw and McKay's research was completed before the era of computers, Bursik and Webb were concerned with testing the cultural transmission hypothesis using more recent data in Chicago and more rigorous quantitative methods. They concluded that the distribution of where delinquents lived in Chicago was not stable from 1950 to 1970 but reflected demographic changes. Variations in delinquency rates in different areas were significantly correlated with variations in the percentage of non-whites, the percentage of foreign-born whites, and the percentage of overcrowded households. The greatest increase in delinquency in an area occurred when blacks moved from the minority to the majority. These results suggest that Shaw and McKay's ideas about community values that persist despite successive waves of immigration and emigration need revising.

The most systematic data available about changes in crime rates over time for larger units than individuals is to be found in official criminal statistics and in repeated victim surveys. These show changes in crime rates for different areas of a country and for whole countries. Unfortunately, these data sources often raise more questions than they answer. For example, the official criminal statistics in the United States and England show that crime has increased dramatically in the last 30 years or so, although there have been some slight decreases in the 1980s. No convincing explanation has yet been proposed for the large increase, which is perhaps the most important criminological phenomenon of all as far as the general public and government agencies are concerned, although it might be related to demographic changes in the population (e.g., Wellford, 1973). Of course, the fact that repeated victim surveys often show little increase in crime enables criminologists to argue that the increase in official statistics was produced artifactually by changes in the way the police and the public reacted to crime.

Attempts have been made to use the official criminal statistics to throw some light on why people commit crimes. For example, one topic of current interest is the effect of unemployment on crime. This has often been studied by correlating official crime rates of a country at different times with official unemployment rates. Unfortunately, this kind of analysis has many problems of interpretation, some caused by measurement problems (e.g., the validity of official measures of crime and unemployment) and some caused by the correlational data. As Tarling (1982) pointed out, since official crime rates have increased over time, anything else that has increased over time—even the consumption of ice cream—will be significantly correlated with them. It is very difficult to disentangle the effects of unemployment from the effects of all the other factors varying over time. Similar problems apply in other analyses based on crime rates—for example, in studies of general deterrence that involve correlating changes in crime rates with changes in the severity or certainty of legal penalties.

The most useful studies based on countries as units are probably the quasi-experimental analyses of new legislation, such as the study of the impact of the breathalyzer test in England by Ross, Campbell, and Glass (1970). (These will be discussed in Chapter 3.) In general, it is probably easier to draw conclusions from longitudinal surveys of smaller units, such as relatively small areas. Few adequate researches of this kind have been carried out. However, the ecological research shows how longitudinal studies of areas can demonstrate continuity or changes in crime rates over time and the extent to which these changes correlate with or seem to follow changes in other factors. These observations can generate causal hypotheses, which, in principle, can be tested experimentally. By collecting data on both individuals and areas over time, it may be possible to disentangle individual and environmental influences. The "ecological fallacy," or the problem of drawing conclusions about individuals from ecological data (Robinson, 1950), might then be laid to rest. More longitudinal studies of areas should be carried out, and Chapter 8 will suggest projects of this kind.

What Have We Learned?

Criminal Careers

As pointed out above, most of the key questions about the explanation, prevention, and treatment of crime can only be answered through detailed knowledge about the course of the development of criminal careers. In reviewing the major findings of longitudinal studies of crime and delinquency, it is logical to begin with knowledge about criminal careers because the greatest contribution of longitudinal studies has been to increase our knowledge about them. We now have a better understanding about what proportion of people commit offenses at different ages, about the numbers and types of crimes committed at different ages, and about when criminal careers begin and end. We also know more about continuity in offending from one age to the next, about specialization or versatility in types of offending, and about the concentration of offending in a small group of "chronic" offenders. Longitudinal studies have also advanced our knowledge about factors that predict the onset or termination of criminal careers, about factors that influence the course of the development of such careers, and about the transmission of offending from one generation to the next.

It is only in recent years that our ways of thinking about criminal careers have become more sophisticated, and the present National Academy of Sciences panel on criminal career research is likely to lead to further conceptual advances. To take what now seems an obvious example, let us return to the fact that officially recorded crime has increased greatly in England and the United States in the last 30 years. Is this because more people are committing crime or because the average offender commits more crimes or both? Unfortunately, the answer to this basic question is not known.

Until recently, much of our knowledge about criminal careers was not only based on official records but also at an aggregate level. In order to make policy recommendations, it is important to disaggregate the data into detailed information about the criminal careers of individuals. For example, cross-sectional data indicate that the peak age for officially recorded crime is in the teens, while the peak age for imprisonment is in the twenties. This led Boland and Wilson (1978) to complain about the inefficiency of a system that most commonly incarcerates people when their criminal activity is low and declining.

The disaggregation of the crime rate (and indeed the imprisonment rate) could show that this complaint might not be warranted. A declining crime rate could reflect a decreasing number of different persons committing crimes, a decreasing number of different types of crime committed by offenders, or a decreasing number of crimes (of any given type) committed by offenders. It is conceivable that the decrease in the overall crime rate with age primarily reflects a decrease in the number of offenders, and that those (relatively few) persons who are still offending are doing so at the same rate as before or even increasing the frequency, diversity, or seriousness of their crimes. It is also conceivable that the residual length of criminal careers could peak at about age 30, for those who continue offending at that age (see Blumstein *et al.*, 1982). Any of these cases could be consistent with the relationship between age and crime seen in the official criminal statistics, but could nevertheless justify a peak age of incarceration (either probability of occurrence or average length of sentence) around age 30. This is not to say that Boland and Wilson's conclusions are wrong, but that they are not necessarily right. This is an example of how conclusions drawn from cross-sectional data might be misleading.

There is a great deal of confusion in the literature regarding such terms as "prevalence" and "incidence." In the interests of clarity, we will use "prevalence" to refer to the proportion of persons who are active offenders at any given time and "cumulative prevalence" to refer to the proportion active up to any given age. "Incidence" will refer to the number of crimes committed by these active offenders. These terms have been explained in more detail by Wilson and Herrnstein (1985, p. 30).

Advances in our ways of thinking about criminal careers limits the usefulness of some of the older longitudinal surveys, such as those by the Gluecks mentioned above. As already pointed out, many of the older surveys were concerned with predicting either delinquency or recidivism, failing to disentangle the different elements of criminal careers. Conceptual and analytic advances mean that it is extremely desirable for raw data collected in longitudinal surveys to be deposited in archives and made available for secondary analyses. The data collected by Wolfgang *et al.* (1972) has already proved very fruitful in this respect [see the section "Secondary Analyses"].

Prevalence Rates at Different Ages

Perhaps because annually published official figures showed a low incidence of offending, it was assumed for many years that crimes were committed by a small deviant minority, even in high-delinquency areas. Theorists were castigated because they predicted "too much" delinquency (see, e.g., Matza, 1964). However, even setting aside the dark figure of undetected crime, longitudinal surveys have shown that when arrests or convictions are cumulated over time, a substantial proportion of the male population is arrested or convicted. In some areas, nonarrested or nonconvicted males are statistically deviant. Longitudinal research is needed to provide cumulative data of this kind.

This surprising finding was first popularized by Wolfgang *et al.* (1972). The cumulative prevalence of nontraffic arrests in their cohort of Philadelphia males was 35% up to age 18 and 47% up to age 30 (Wolfgang, 1983). However, this was not really a new result. Fifteen years earlier, the longitudinal survey of Hathaway and Monachesi (1957) had reported that 41% of Minneapolis boys had their names in police records for some kind of crime by age 19. Of course, there are problems in using arrests as measures of criminal behavior. Many arrests do not lead to convictions, in some cases because of legal technicalities but in other cases because the persons arrested are innocent.

As the detailed review by Gordon (1976) shows, the cumulative prevalence of crime varies a great deal with different definitions. This is brought out very clearly in the work of Shannon (1981) in Racine, Wisconsin. He studied three birth cohorts, born in 1942, 1949, and 1955, followed up in records to ages 33, 26, and 21, respectively. Of the males in the three cohorts, 84%, 82%, and 72%, respectively, had a recorded police contact of some kind. The corresponding figures for the females were 48%, 52%, and 45%. However, the proportions with contacts for relatively serious offenses (felonies and major misdemeanors, which might be considered "real crimes") were 22%, 23%, and 23% for the males and 2%, 5%, and 6% for the females.

The cumulative prevalence of police contacts of males is also high in other countries, as shown by two large studies in Copenhagen. Wolf (1984) in the Danish *Project Metropolitan* reported that 35% of 12,270 boys born in 1953 had been registered by the police for at least one offense committed before age 23. Similarly, Guttridge, Gabrielli, Mednick, and Van Dusen (1983) found that 38% of 28,879 boys born during 1944 and 1947 had been arrested by age 27–30. Unfortunately, these two percentages include traffic offenses. According to Wolf (personal communication), 21% of his cohort were registered for nontraffic offenses.

In the London cohort of Farrington (1983b), about one-third were convicted for a criminal (nontraffic) offense up to the twenty-fifth birthday. Unlike the United States, arrests in London were in most cases followed by convictions. The peak age for the number of different youths convicted was 17, with 12% convicted at that age alone. The peak age for most types of offenses was about 17, but it was earlier for shoplifting and theft from automatic machines and later for assault, damage, drug use, and fraud. In the Philadelphia cohort study, the peak age for the prevalence of arrests was 16 (Collins, 1981).

An important question concerns the influence of jurisdictional ages on prevalence rates. In England, it is noticeable that the peak age of 17 is also the minimum age for adult court. It could be that police officers are inhibited from taking young persons to court as long as they are legally juveniles but lose these inhibitions when the young people become legally adults. It would be interesting to carry out a systematic comparison of prevalence rates between states of the United States (or provinces of Canada) with minimum ages for adult court of 16 or 17 and those with minimum ages of 18. Ruhland, Gold, and Hekman (1982) did something like this in investigating the general deterrent effects of adult as opposed to juvenile court. Since they found that 17-year-olds admitted more offenses in states where they were juveniles than in states where they were adults, they concluded that the adult court had a greater general deterrent effect.

Little is known about the cumulative prevalence rate of offenses that do not necessarily result in police contacts. More is known about the prevalence rate at different ages. The most detailed figures are those obtained in the Elliott survey (Elliott, Ageton, Huizinga, Knowles, and Canter, 1983; Elliott and Huizinga, 1983; Ageton, 1983). They used "prevalence" to refer to the proportion of people who committed at least one offense in one year and "incidence" to refer to the average number of offenses committed per person (not per offender) in that year. As usual, the results depend a great deal on the definition of delinquency. For example, using a wide definition (their "general delinquency B"), about two-thirds of young people committed at least one delinquent act in a year. However, only about 1 in 6 committed an index offense in a year. (Note: Index, or Part I, offenses in the FBI statistics consist of murder, forcible rape, robbery, aggravated assault, burglary, theft, motor vehicle theft, and arson.)

It is difficult to interpret the prevalence rates at different ages published by Elliott *et al.* (1983) because of the marked decline from 1976 (when 21% admitted an index offense) to 1980 (when the corresponding figure was only 12%). These figures might reflect a real decline in offending over time, or rather, effects of testing such that the young people became successively less willing to admit offenses over time. Also, their figures seem to be subject to a great deal of sampling variability. Restricting the analysis to ages with at least three estimates from different cohorts, the peak age for the prevalence of index offenses was 15 to 17 (with 18% of the sample committing at least one index offense at each of these ages). A multiple cohort longitudinal survey such as this does allow the possibility of disentangling changes with age from changes with period. As an example of this, Elliott, Knowles, and Canter (1981) compared their figures with the earlier data of Gold and Reimer (1975), and showed that the proportion of 13 to 16-year-olds committing delinquent acts had increased between 1967 and 1977.

Farrington (1983b) also provided self-report information about prevalence rates at each age. As he found with official convictions, the peak age for most offenses was between 15 and 18. During these three years, 62% of the males were involved in fights, 32% used drugs, 21% damaged property, 15% took vehicles, 13% stole from vehicles, and 11% committed at least one burglary. The peak age for shoplifting, however, was clearly earlier. The conviction records and self-reports agreed substantially in identifying the most serious offenders. For example, between ages 15 and 18, 11% were identified as burglars by self-report, 7% by conviction records, and 5% by both.

Estimating the prevalence rate for different types of crimes at different ages is, to a considerable extent, only a first step in understanding criminal behavior. Nevertheless, it is an important one. The next step is to investigate changes in other factors or life events that predict or correlate with changes in prevalence. We will return to this in the section "Onset, Duration, and Termination" in discussing predictors of the onset and termination of offending careers.

Incidence Rates at Different Ages

The clearest distinctions between different aspects of criminal careers have been made by Blumstein (e.g., Blumstein and Cohen, 1979; Blumstein *et al.*, 1982).

He has popularized the use of the term "individual crime rate" at each age, or the number of offenses committed per offender, and has emphasized the importance of distinguishing this from the prevalence rate. We prefer to refer to the individual crime rate as the "incidence." In most surveys, it is difficult to know whether changes in overall crime rates per sample member reflect changes in prevalence or in incidence. For example, Shannon (1981) showed that the peak age for the average number of police contacts per cohort member was 16–17 for males and 17–19 for females, but whether these peaks primarily reflect prevalence or incidence is not clear. As was pointed out in the section "Criminal Careers," in evaluating penal policy options it is often crucially important to be able to disentangle these quantities.

It is possible to calculate incidence rates from the data given by Elliott *et al.* (1981) because they provide both the prevalence and the average rate of offending for the whole sample. For example, in 1976, 21% of the sample committed index offenses, and the average number committed per sample member was 1.01. It therefore follows that the average number of index offenses committed per offender was 4.8 (1.01/.21). According to our calculations, there was no clear tendency for the incidence of offending to vary with age.

Farrington (1983a) calculated both prevalence and incidence for official and self-reported offenses. The incidence did not vary with age in the same way as the prevalence. In the case of convictions, this was because most convicted persons were only convicted once during each age range. In the case of self-reported offenses, incidence rates sometimes decreased after age 18 as the prevalence rate decreased (e.g., with fighting and burglary); but on other occasions (e.g., damage and stealing from vehicles), a decrease in the prevalence rate after age 18 coincided with an increase in the incidence rate. It seems likely that the well-known peak age of offending reflects a peak in prevalence rather than incidence.

An important question is the extent to which incidence rates can be predicted. This was addressed in a retrospective self-report survey of prisoners by Greenwood and Abrahamse (1982). They found remarkable variations in offending rates, from low-rate offenders committing only one or two offenses per year to high-rate offenders committing hundreds. They proposed a method of predicting the high-rate offenders in advance, based on such factors as prior criminal history, juvenile record, and a history of drug use. Greenwood and Abrahamse argued that incarceration should be used more selectively: predicted high-rate offenders should receive longer prison sentences, while predicted low-rate offenders should receive shorter ones (or noncustodial sentences). If a penal policy of this kind was adopted, they estimated that, in California, it would be possible to achieve a 15% reduction in the robbery rate together with a 5% reduction in the incarcerated population.

This kind of policy option is likely to prove very attractive to legislators, prosecutors, and judges. Previous incapacitation research on the effects of mandatory sentences has involved impractically large increases in prison populations. For example, the mandatory five-year sentences for felony convictions considered by Petersilia and Greenwood (1978) would have led to a prison population increase of 450%. The promise that a policy of selective incapacitation might allow a decrease in the crime rate together with no increase in the incarcerated population seems too good to be true. Unfortunately, it may be. In studying the prediction of incidence rates, the prediction research of Greenwood and Abrahamse represents a great step forward. However, it still suffers from many of the problems ignored by the Gluecks (1950) more than 30 years before. For example, Greenwood and Abrahamse's research was entirely retrospective and had no validation sample. Before a policy of selective incapacitation is brought into effect, it is essential that their results should be replicated in a prospective longitudinal survey.

From the point of view of assessing penal aims such as deterrence and incapacitation, it is desirable to establish not only the prevalence and incidence at each age, but also the probability of an arrest following an offense, the probability of a conviction following an arrest, the probability of an incarceration following a conviction, and the average time served in each incarceration. Little is known about how these quantities vary with age in cohorts. However, Peterson, Braiker, and Polich (1981) studied changes in arrest probabilities with age in a cross-sectional survey of California prison inmates and found no clear trends. In the London longitudinal survey, Langan and Farrington (1983) were able to calculate the probability of a conviction leading to incarceration at different ages. While this probability was highest at the latest age studied (23–24), it did not increase steadily but in fact fluctuated over the whole age range from 10 to 24. When sentence length was taken into account, it emerged that the average length of time incarcerated following a conviction was highest at ages 23–24 but second highest at age 14. More research of this kind is needed.

Onset, Duration, and Termination

Longitudinal surveys can provide information about when offending begins, about how long it lasts, and about when it ends. Cross-sectional surveys usually cannot provide this information, which is important for penal policy. For example, attempts to prevent crime could concentrate on the period just before the age of onset. Also, from the viewpoint of incapacitation, there would be little point in extending a prison sentence beyond the age of termination.

Information about the cumulative probability of a first arrest for index offenses was provided in the survey by Wolfgang et al. (1972). This probability began at a low level at age 7, increased to a maximum rate of increase at age 15, and thereafter the rate of increase slowed down. The peak age of onset of index arrests was 15. In the survey by Farrington (1983b), the peak age of onset of convictions was between 13 and 15, while the peak age for the number of convictions was between 14 and 20. Little is known about the age of onset of offenses not leading to official action. However, Elliott and Huizinga (1984) published figures from their longitudinal survey showing the percentage of persons initiating offenses at each age, and found that initiation peaked at 13–15.

Little is known about the distribution of ages of termination of offending. Polk *et al.* (1981) produced a distribution of the year of the last arrest for their sample, for men with no arrests in the last three years of their project (ages 27–30). This peaked in 1966 (at age 17, presumably). Elliott and Huizinga (1984) also showed the percentage of persons terminating at each age, finding that this peaked at 18–19. However, in this important self-report survey, it is difficult to be sure that all initiations and terminations are genuine, in view of the limited period covered (five annual interviews). Barnett and Lofaso (1985) could find no evidence of termination of offending up to the eighteenth birthday in the Philadelphia cohort. Virtually all the apparent termination was "false desistence" caused by the truncation of the data at age 18.

Of course, until a person has died, it is difficult to be sure that their offending has terminated. Even a 10-year conviction-free period is no guarantee of this, as longitudinal surveys have shown. For example, Gibbens (1984) followed up a sample of 199 borstal boys in records for 25 years after conviction. After 10 years, 43 were not reconvicted, but 13 of these were convicted subsequently. It would be desirable for researchers with older samples (e.g., McCord, 1979) to attempt to map out ages of termination for different types of offense and offending careers.

It would also be desirable for researchers to investigate the distribution of lengths of criminal careers and the expected residual length at any given age. It is known that an early age of onset of offending is generally followed by a long career. For example, Farrington (1983a) showed that the average conviction career length was greatest for those first convicted at ages 10–12. Career length was measured by the time between the first and last conviction, and it averaged 8.2 years for these early convicted boys. However, this analysis only included convictions up to the twenty-fifth birthday. The early convicted boys averaged more convictions per year during their careers than any other group, suggesting that their incidence rates were higher. One practical implication of this result is that there is a considerable potential for reducing crime by concentrating on those who offend at the youngest ages.

Somewhat similar conclusions were reached by Hamparian, Schuster, Dinitz, and Conrad (1978) and Miller *et al.* (1982) with their violent offenders. Those arrested at the earliest ages had the largest total number of arrests. However, after the age of onset, the rate of official offending was tolerably constant over time. Loeber (1982) reviewed several studies on age of onset and identified the ages of 7–11 as particularly significant. The onset of offending at this age was associated with more delinquent or criminal activity in total, more serious acts, and a higher rate of offending. The first arrest was usually preceded by high rates of antisocial behavior in school, in the family home, and in the neighborhood. Whether these results would hold up with self-report measures of offending or of the onset age is not clear.

Quite a number of longitudinal surveys have been concerned with predicting which people become offenders out of an initial sample of nonoffenders (i.e., predicting onset as opposed to the age at onset). As pointed out earlier in the section "Desirable Features of Longitudinal Surveys," the prediction of delinquency or recidivism has probably been the major concern of past longitudinal researchers, from the Gluecks (1930) onward. It is worthwhile restating the predictors of onset in the important research of McCord (1979). She concluded that (a) poor parental supervision and the mother's lack of self-confidence predicted convictions for property and personal crimes, (b) the mother's lack of affection and the father's deviance (alcoholism or conviction for a serious crime) predicted property but not personal crimes, and (c) parental conflict and parental aggression (e.g., beating children) predicted personal but not property crimes.

West and Farrington (1973) found that a large number of factors measured before age 10 were predictive of future convictions, particularly troublesome behavior at the primary school, low family income, large family size, convicted parents, low IQ, and poor parental child-rearing behavior (a combination of cruel or neglecting attitudes, harsh or erratic discipline, and parental conflict). In general, convictions and self-reported offending were quite closely related, so that the predictors of convictions tended also to predict self-reported offending. However, there were some differences. For example, whereas convicted parents predicted both, low family income was a better predictor of convictions than of self-reported offending. This result suggests that low family income may be related to the likelihood of being selected for official processing rather than to the likelihood of committing offenses.

Loeber and Dishion (1983) have carried out a detailed review of (mostly longitudinal) studies of the prediction of delinquency and of recidivism. It might be thought that the prediction of recidivism is the reverse of the prediction of termination of offending, but this depends on the length of the follow-up period. In other words, the absence of recidivism does not necessarily indicate termination. Throughout all the studies, they found that the best predictors of delinquency (i.e., onset) were parental family management techniques, followed by the child's own antisocial behavior, criminal or antisocial behavior of other family members, and the child's poor educational achievement. The predictors of recidivism were somewhat different. The best predictors were the child's own antisocial or delinquent behavior and the criminal or antisocial behavior of other family members. It is perhaps not surprising that parental family management techniques should be important in relation to onset but not to termination because children are much more likely to be affected by the control of their parents at the time of onset. On the other hand, parental family-management techniques have not been measured in many recidivism studies because such studies are usually based only on factors available in official records.

A series of explicit attempts to predict the termination of conviction careers was carried out in the Cambridge Study in Delinquent Development (Knight and West, 1975; Osborn and West, 1978, 1980). The aim was to predict, out of those with two or more convictions before age 19, those who would be convicted again during the next five years. As might have been expected, the most obvious difference between the "persisters" and the "terminators" was that the persisters had more extensive prior conviction records. Persisters were also more likely to come from large, low-income families, and to have convicted parents. Furthermore, they were rated as more "antisocial" at age 18, in displaying a variety of behaviors such as sexual promiscuity, heavy gambling and smoking, driving after drinking, and aggression. These results show the lasting predictive power of some of the earliest life experiences and the importance of later deviant life-styles.

As is true in other sections, longitudinal research has advanced our knowledge of the onset, duration, and termination of offending careers, and of the predictors of onset and termination, but it has also drawn attention to gaps in our knowledge. The information about prediction is useful as a first step in formulating explanations of why such careers begin and end. Some explanations proposed by longitudinal researchers will be reviewed in the section "Implications for Criminological Theories."

Continuity in Offending

An advantage of longitudinal research is its ability to link up offending at one stage of a criminal career with offending at another. Thus, it is possible to specify what proportion of juvenile offenders become adult ones and vice versa. It is also possible to establish the probability of one offense being followed by another and the extent to which offenders tend to specialize in certain types of crimes or switch from one to another.

The relation between juvenile and adult offending has important policy implications. If most people "grow out" of juvenile crime and do not commit offenses as adults (as seems to be widely believed), then it may not be necessary to arrest and convict to many juvenile offenders. This argument becomes especially forceful when combined with evidence (Gold, 1970; Farrington, 1977; Miller and Gold, 1984) that official processing of juveniles tends to lead to an increase rather than a decrease in delinquent behavior (see Chapter 5). On the other hand, if the majority of adult offenders had previously been juvenile ones, then it may be more important to try to prevent crime in the future by taking action when people are still young. In the United States, juvenile records are not often used in the adult courts, leading Boland and Wilson (1978) to argue that this "two-track" system of justice was inequitable and provided inefficient protection for the general public. A former chronic juvenile delinquent appearing in the adult court for the first time was likely to be sentenced erroneously as a first offender (see Langan and Farrington, 1983).

Longitudinal surveys show a marked relationship between juvenile and adult arrests. Because of the widespread failure to link up juvenile with adult records, and the destruction or sealing of juvenile records, this relationship is difficult to study retrospectively using official data. In the Philadelphia cohort study, Wolfgang (1980) found that 39% of those arrested as juveniles were also arrested as adults (up to age 30), compared with 9% of those not arrested as juveniles. Conversely, 69% of those arrested as adults had been arrested as juveniles, compared with 25% of those not arrested as adults. In the Oregon study by Polk *et al.* (1981), 49% of those arrested as juveniles were also arrested as adults (up to age 30), compared with 22% of those not arrested as juveniles. Conversely, 38% of those arrested as adults had been arrested as juveniles, compared with 13% of those not arrested as adults. The precise figures differ according to the overall proportions arrested as juveniles and as adults, but the marked relationship is obvious in both studies.

Other longitudinal surveys have also provided useful information about the relationship between officially recorded juvenile delinquency and adult crime. In the longest follow-up by McCord (1979), beyond age 45, nearly half (47%) of those convicted of serious crimes as juveniles were similarly convicted as adults, in comparison with 18% of those not convicted as juveniles. Conversely, 42% of those convicted as adults had also been convicted as juveniles, in comparison with 15% of those not convicted as adults. Similar relationships between juvenile and adult crime are seen in the three cohorts of Shannon (1981).

One problem with these results is the argument that the continuity between juvenile and adult arrests reflects continuity in police activity rather than in offending, as it is likely that police attention and suspicion are especially focused on persons with previous criminal records. Farrington (1983a) showed a strong relationship in England between juvenile and adult conviction records. However, he was able also to demonstrate a strong relationship between juvenile and adult self-reported offending, even among unconvicted persons. These findings suggest that there is continuity in offending.

Whether juvenile delinquency leads to adult crime is part of a more general question about the probability of one offense leading to another, at different ages. One of the important contributions of the longitudinal survey of Wolfgang *et al.* (1972) was to calculate these probabilities. For all nontraffic offenses, the probability of a first arrest was .35, of a second following a first was .54, and of a third following a second was .65. This probability hovered around the .72 level for the next three transitions and then rose to about .80 for the probability of a seventh arrest onward. Wolfgang and Tracy (1982) then repeated this analysis for the males in their second cohort (born in 1958), with similar results. The probability of a first arrest was .33, of a second following a first was .58, and this probability increased to around .80 for transitions after the fifth. The high probabilities for the later transitions suggest that there is a group of unusually persistent or "chronic" offenders and these will be considered further in the section "The Chronic Offenders."

Several other researchers have calculated these recidivism probabilities, always finding the same pattern of increases. For example, Polk *et al.* (1981) also studied juvenile nontraffic arrests of males. The probability of a first offense was .25, of a second following a first was .47, of a third following a second was .58, and this gradually rose to about .74 for arrests after the fifth. In the Shannon (1981) study, the prevalence of a first nontraffic police contact was high. For example, it was .70 in the 1942 cohort for males up to age 33. However, even with this high starting value, the probability rose to about .88 for contacts after the fifth. The same pattern was found in the English research of Farrington (1983b).

For nontraffic convictions of males up to the twenty-fifth birthday, the probability of a first offense was .33, of a second following a first .63, and this rose to about .87 for convictions after the sixth.

Another surprising result first highlighted by Wolfgang *et al.* (1972) was the lack of specialization in juvenile offending. When offenses were divided into five broad types (nonindex, injury, theft, damage, and combination), it was found that the type of offense committed on any arrest did not relate to the type committed on the previous arrest. It seemed that offenders committed types of offenses at random rather than specializing in theft or damage or whatever. A complete lack of specialization, however, is unusual. It is more usual to find some specialization superimposed on a high degree of generality. For example, Wolfgang (1980) reported that there was evidence of specialization in his adult data. Similarly, in retrospective surveys by Bursik (1980) and Rojek and Erickson (1982) there was some evidence of specialization, although a high degree of generality. Self-reported offending also shows versatility (e.g., Hindelang, 1971; Farrington, 1973; Peterson *et al.*, 1981), although offense-to-offense transition matrices for it have not yet been published. The most extensive review of the topic of versatility versus specialization in juvenile offending has been provided by Klein (1984), who concluded that it was predominantly versatile.

Another important result obtained in the Wolfgang *et al.* (1972) survey was that the average seriousness of juvenile offenses increased somewhat with age. The average seriousness of adult offenses increased much more steeply with age (Wolfgang, 1980). Similarly, the average seriousness of juvenile offenses increased at each successive arrest, while the average seriousness of adult offenses increased more steeply at each successive arrest. It is important to try to measure the quality of offenses as well as their legal categories.

Offenders are not only versatile in committing different types of offenses but also in committing different kinds of other deviant acts. For example, West and Farrington (1977) found that their convicted youths at age 18 drank more beer, got drunk more often, and were more likely to say that drink made them violent than the nonconvicted youths. The convicted youths smoked more cigarettes, had started smoking at an earlier age, and were more likely to be heavy gamblers. They were more likely to have been found guilty of minor motoring offenses, to have driven after drinking at least five pints of beer, and to have been injured in road accidents. They were more likely to have taken prohibited drugs such as marijuana or LSD, even though very few were convicted for this. They were also more likely to have had sexual intercourse with a variety of different girls, especially beginning at an early age, but they were less likely than the remainder to use contraceptives. In many respects, the types of deviant acts that attracted police attention were only one aspect of a larger syndrome of deviant or antisocial behavior. This result draws attention to the limitations of research based on official criminal records. Such research will miss the continuities between criminal offenses and other kinds of deviant acts.

Longitudinal surveys can also investigate developmental sequences or the extent to which one kind of deviant act or offense leads to another. One of the most interesting studies on this topic was carried by Robins and Wish (1977).

They distinguished between quantitative developmental processes, where the likelihood of committing an untried deviant act depended principally on the number of other types of acts already tried, and qualitative processes, where certain specific acts tended to be stepping stones to others. They studied 13 acts of childhood (before age 18) deviance, including elementary school failure and truancy, dropping out of high school before graduation, juvenile arrests, precocious sexual experience, drinking, and drug use, in their sample of 223 black males in St. Louis.

In general, all the acts tended to be related to each other, reflecting the versatility of deviant behavior. However, the acts that were closest in age of onset tended to be most closely related. Few significant relationships between one act and a later one held independently of the number of acts committed before the first one. This suggested that the developmental process was primarily quantitative (versatile) rather than qualitative (specialized). The likelihood of an act being committed in the future depended on the *number* of acts committed in the past, rather than on the types of acts committed. However, there were some qualitative relationships that were plausible theoretically. For example, drinking led to marijuana and amphetamine use, truancy led to dropping out of school, and (in the only reciprocal relationship) truancy led to school failure and school failure led to truancy.

Robins and Ratcliff (1980) then investigated the relationship between nine types of childhood deviant acts and five types of adult arrests. In general, the probability of an adult arrest increased with the number of different types of childhood deviance. They went on the study whether specific types of childhood deviant acts predicted specific types of adult arrests, controling both for the number of childhood deviant acts and for the number of adult arrests. The only significant relationship was in drug use. For sex, the relationship was opposite to the expected one because those with early sex experience were less likely to commit rape than the remainder. Robins has consistently argued that since the major relationships in her research are quantitative rather than qualitative (the overall level of childhood deviance predicting the overall level of adult deviance), there is a single syndrome made up of a broad variety of antisocial acts arising in childhood and continuing into adulthood. The continuity between antisocial and criminal behavior suggests that preventive action in childhood, even if aimed at acts that are deviant rather than delinquent, might be beneficial in reducing adult offending.

The Chronic Offenders

One of the most famous results obtained by Wolfgang *et al.* (1972) was that a small proportion of their cohort (the chronic offenders, defined as those with five or more arrests) accounted for a large proportion of the offenses. In their first cohort, the 6% of the sample who were chronics accounted for 52% of all juvenile arrests. In their second cohort, the 7% who were chronics accounted for 61% of all juvenile arrests (Wolfgang and Tracy, 1982). Similar results have been obtained by other researchers. For example, Shannon (1981) reported that 6% of his third cohort were responsible for 51% of all police contacts up to age 21. In England, Farrington (1983b) found that 6% of his sample accounted not only for 49% of all the convictions up to the twenty-fifth birthday, but also for substantial proportions of the self-reported offenses. Also, in a national sample of English males born in 1953, the 5.5% who each had six or more convictions were responsible for 70% of all convictions up to age 28 (Home Office, 1985).

This concentration of offending can best be shown in longitudinal research in which crimes are cumulated over time. The demonstration of the chronic offenders has been an important factor in the development of career criminal prosecution programs in many jurisdictions of the United States. These aim to concentrate prosecution resources on serious, repeat offenders, to increase their conviction rates and average periods of incarceration (see, e.g., Greenwood, 1980). As mentioned elsewhere, it is believed that selective incapacitation of chronic offenders may lead to a significant reduction in the crime rate.

A recent objection to these ideas has come from Dunford and Elliott (1984). They were concerned with identifying the high-rate, persistent offenders using their longitudinal self-report data. They defined "serious career offenders" as those committing at least 3 index offenses in at least two consecutive years out of the five studied, and "nonserious career offenders" as others committing at least 12 delinquent acts in at least two consecutive years. They had arrest data for three years only, and showed that the six youths with five or more arrests all fell into this classification of career offenders. However, out of 242 self-reported career offenders, 86% had no arrest record, 12% had 1–4 arrests, and only 2% had 5 or more arrests. Therefore, "defining career offenders in terms of youth with five or more arrests means that all but a tiny fraction of youth engaged in frequent and serious offending will be overlooked" (p. 79).

There are a number of problems with this argument. First of all, the "index offenses" admitted might not be regarded as such by the police. The most common one was gang fights, and others included strong-arming students and teachers. Similarly, the "delinquent" acts, which included hitting teachers, parents, and students, might not have led to arrests even if they had been detected by the police. The grouping together of serious and nonserious career offenders muddies the water a little. About a quarter of the serious career offenders were arrested in one of the three years, in comparison with only 10% of the nonserious career offenders. Second, given that 27% of the target sample was not interviewed in the first round of data collection, the most persistent and serious offenders in the population may have been underrepresented in their sample. Their serious career offenders seem unlikely to be comparable in seriousness of offending to the inner-city Philadelphia chronics.

Third, the police arrest data may be incomplete. The searches only included juveniles who consented to have their records searched (88% of those interviewed) and only covered jurisdictions within 10 miles of a juvenile's home. Also, the arrest records extended over three years only (1976–78), rather than covering the complete juvenile history. A person who committed three or more index offenses only in 1979 and 1980 and who was arrested only in both of those years would be classified as a nonarrested serious career offender. We could not agree with the above quotation without seeing both self-report and official data covering much longer periods, and perhaps with the self-report data restricted to clear index offenses such as theft of motor vehicles, robbery, and burglary.

More fundamental objections to the concept of chronic offenders have been put forward by Blumstein and Moitra (1980). First of all, they pointed out that the most appropriate figure was not the 6% of the Wolfgang *et al.* cohort but the 18% of the offenders who accounted for 52% of the arrests. After all, 35% of the cohort accounted for 100% of the arrests, but this disproportionality was not considered surprising. Second, the chronics were identified retrospectively rather than prospectively. Even if all the arrested boys had the same probability of recidivism constant over time, chance factors alone would result in some of them having more arrests and others fewer. Of course, those with the most arrests would account for a disproportionate fraction of the total number of arrests.

Blumstein and Moitra went on to investigate how far it was possible to fit the data of Wolfgang *et al.* with the assumption that the chronics did not differ from less serious offenders in rearrest probabilities. They showed that the data could be fitted by dividing the offenders into the "amateurs" with one or two arrests and the "persisters" with three or more. This model showed how those with five or more arrests could account for the majority of the arrests even when they were indistinguishable in rearrest probability from those with three or four arrests. As they pointed out, the important question left unanswered in the Philadelphia data was whether the chronics could be identified in advance.

Blumstein, Farrington, and Moitra (1985) then investigated the extent to which chronic offenders in the London cohort study could be identified in advance. They assumed that there were two subpopulations of convicted youths: the persisters, with a high recidivism probability, and the desisters, with a low recidivism probability. Because of chance processes, the desisters soon dropped out of the offending population, which came to be increasingly composed of persisters. To a considerable extent, the "chronics" with six or more convictions could be predicted at the time of the first conviction. A prediction score was developed based on poor school behavior, economic deprivation, convicted parents, low intelligence, and poor parental child-rearing behavior. The results obtained by using this prediction score to classify boys as persisters or desisters at the time of the first conviction agreed quite well with those expected on the theoretical model of persisters and desisters and with the actual distribution of convictions observed.

The implications of these analyses are that chronics (defined retrospectively according to a certain number of observed arrests) cannot be identified in advance as well as persisters (defined according to a high probability of recidivism) can be. These longitudinal analyses enable us to have a more appropriate way of thinking about this prediction problem.

Intergenerational Transmission

Longitudinal research is useful in investigating the transmission of criminal behavior from one generation to the next. Ideally, such a study should begin with one generation and follow the next generation of their children from birth onward. One of the few projects to have followed two successive generations from the birth of the first one is the British National Survey (Wadsworth, 1979). Efforts have been made to collect comparable information about both generations, but little data on the transmission of criminal behavior has yet emerged.

In the United States, Robins *et al.* (1975) and McCord (1977) have attempted to study intergenerational transmission. Robins *et al.* compared male and female children with their fathers and mothers, the fathers being the black men referred to earlier. In general, arrested parents tended to have arrested children, and the juvenile records of the parents and children showed similar rates and types of offenses. McCord found that convicted sons (her subjects) tended to have convicted fathers. Whether there is a specific relationship between types of convictions of parents and children is not clear. McCord reported that 29% of fathers convicted for violence had sons convicted for violence, in comparison with 12% of other fathers, but this may reflect the general tendency for convicted fathers to have convicted sons rather than any specific tendency for violent fathers to have violent sons.

In their English study, West and Farrington (1977) showed that convicted fathers and mothers tended to have convicted children. However, because they interviewed both parents and children, they were able to investigate some possible reasons for this transmission. There was no indication that convicted fathers directly encouraged their sons to commit crimes or taught them criminal techniques. The major difference between convicted and unconvicted fathers was that the convicted fathers exercised poorer supervision over their sons. There was some evidence that the sons of criminal fathers were more likely to be convicted over and above their increased likelihood of committing delinquent acts (as measured by self-reports). It may be that, when the police catch a youth committing an offense and know that he comes from a family containing other convicted persons, they are more likely to prosecute and secure a conviction than in other cases. This factor, and the poor supervision, were the major links West and Farrington could find in the chain between convicted parents and convicted children.

One possible reason why convicted parents have convicted children may be because some factor connected with criminal behavior is transmitted genetically. Several Scandinavian longitudinal surveys have been designed to investigate this possibility. Three broad methods have been used, namely, following up identical and fraternal twins, following up adopted children, and following up children with specific genetic abnormalities.

The basic idea underlying twin studies is that identical and fraternal twins both have the same environment from birth. However, identical twins are more similar in heredity than fraternal ones. Therefore, if identical twins are more similar in their criminal history than fraternal ones, this is taken as evidence for some kind of hereditary influence on crime. The largest twin study was carried out by Christiansen (1968, 1974). He followed up all (3,600) twin pairs born in Denmark during 1881–1910 where both twins survived at least until age 15, the age of criminal responsibility. He found that when one twin had been convicted, the other was much more likely to have also been convicted if they were identical twins than if they were fraternal ones. This result suggests a hereditary component in criminal behavior.

The major objection to twin studies is that identical twins may have a more identical environment than fraternal ones because they tend to be treated more identically. Hence, the greater similarity of identical twins in criminal behavior may reflect not genetic but environmental influences. Some evidence relevant to this argument was obtained by Dalgard and Kringlen (1976). They followed up all male twins born in Norway during 1921–1930 and tried to interview and obtain blood tests (for zygosity determination) from pairs containing at least one person convicted. They found that identical twins were more similar in convictions than fraternal ones. However, whether the twins had a subjective feeling of closeness and mutual identity was more important than whether they were identical or fraternal. Fraternal twins who felt similar to each other were just as similar in their criminal records as identical twins who felt similar. Dalgard and Kringlen concluded that similarity in environmental treatment mattered more than similarity in heredity. However, it is impossible to be sure in their research that the similarity in feelings preceded the criminal behavior. It could be that, when two members of a twin pair were convicted, this caused them to feel more similar. As usual, prospective longitudinal research is needed to unravel the question of order.

The most conclusive twin studies are those in which identical and fraternal twins were separated at birth. For example, in a small scale study Shields (1962) showed that identical twins brought up apart were no less similar in intelligence and personality than those brought up together, suggesting that genetic factors were important in both intelligence and personality. However, the separated twin method has not yet been used to study genetic factors in crime.

Moving on to adoption studies, the most famous was carried out by Mednick, Gabrielli, and Hutchings (1983). They followed up all (14,400) persons born in Denmark from 1924 to 1947 and adopted by someone outside the biological family. They compared the conviction records of the adoptees with those of their biological and adoptive parents. They found that convictions of sons were significantly related to convictions of biological parents but not to convictions of adoptive parents. This suggests again that there is some kind of hereditary factor in crime. Mednick et al. also considered a number of possible nongenetic explanations for their results. In particular, their findings were not affected by the age at which the boy was adopted (mostly soon after birth). Against the theory that their results reflected the labeling of children with convicted biological parents, the conclusions held independently of whether the parent was convicted before or after the boy's birth.

The most extensive relevant American adoption study is probably that by Cadoret and Cain (1980) in Iowa. From adoption records between 1939 and 1965, attempts were made to locate adoptees who were separated from their biological parents at birth, who had no contact with their biological family, who were placed in a permanent adoptive home, and whose biological parent had a psychiatric condition. A similar group of adoptees was located where neither parent had a psychiatric condition, and both groups were interviewed by someone who did not know which group they were in. Cadoret and Cain found that antisocial behavior in the children (including getting into trouble with police or courts) was predicted by having an alcoholic or antisocial biological parent. As with many psychiatric studies, criminal behavior was not studied separately from other kinds of deviance.

Finally, as an example of a follow-up of specific genetic abnormalities, Witkin *et al.* (1976) tried to investigate the relationship between XXY and XYY chromosome abnormalities and convictions. They followed up all males born in Copenhagen between 1944 and 1947. The Danish national register provided their addresses at age 26, and the draft boards, to which all men were required to report by age 26, provided information about their adult heights. The two abnormalities were known to be more prevalent among tall men. More than 4,500 men with heights exceeding 6 feet were identified, and attempts were made to visit every one of them to take blood samples and buccal smears to determine chromosomal constitution. This determination was made successfully in 91% of cases, but unfortunately only 16 XXY and 12 XYY males were found. The XYY males were particularly likely to have been convicted, but conclusions are of course limited by the small numbers.

It can be seen that there are some tentative indications of a hereditary factor in criminal behavior, but the precise nature of this factor is unknown. What is needed are longitudinal studies of the transmission of criminal behavior in which the characteristics of the criminal careers of the parents and children are measured more carefully. In particular, are parents and children similar in incidence rates, types of offenses committed, ages of onset and termination, and duration of careers? Are similar results obtained with official and self-report measures? It would be sensible to establish some of these basic results before embarking on difficult and costly biological determinations.

Effects of Events on Development

With the exception of a few experiments on the effects of penal treatments, which will be reviewed in Chapter 3, few criminological researchers have taken advantage of the potentialities of longitudinal surveys in investigating the effects of specific events on the course of development of criminal careers. This is surprising because if it could be shown that the occurrence of a specific event (e.g., the onset of unemployment) was reliably followed by a change in criminal behavior, this would suggest a causal relationship. Most longitudinal researchers are still essentially analyzing their data as though it was obtained cross-sectionally, relying on statistical control of extraneous variables. A quasi-experimental analysis would be better, and a randomized experiment better still, from the point of view of drawing conclusions about what influences criminal careers. Both of these approaches will be discussed more fully in Chapter 3.

As examples of how longitudinal data could be analyzed to investigate the effects of specific events, three studies carried out with the London cohort will be described. The first was concerned with the effects of convictions on delinquent behavior. If convictions have some kind of individual deterrent or rehabilitative effects, it might be expected that delinquent behavior would decrease after they occur. On the other hand, if convictions have some kind of stigmatizing or labeling effects, delinquent behavior might increase after them. In studying the effects of convictions longitudinally, Farrington (1977) investigated self-reported offending at ages 14 and 18 for boys convicted for the first time between these ages and for unconvicted boys matched at age 14. The convicted boys significantly increased their offending by the later age. Similar results were obtained for first convictions between 18 and 21 (Farrington *et al.*, 1978). After testing plausible alternative explanations of the results, it was concluded that the convictions produced an increase in offending (see also Chapter 5).

The second study investigated the effects on offending of going to different secondary schools (Farrington, 1972). Again, this essentially took advantage of the before-and-after measures available in the longitudinal survey. As might have been expected, boys going to high-delinquency-rate secondary schools at 11 were more likely to be convicted than those going to low-delinquency-rate schools. However, the differing prevalence of convictions between the secondary schools could be largely explained by their differing intakes. Generally, the high-delinquency-rate secondary schools received boys who had been troublesome in their primary schools, with a high likelihood of future convictions, while the low-delinquency-rate secondary schools received well-behaved boys. It seemed that the schools themselves had relatively little effect on delinquency (but see Chapter 4).

The third study investigated the effects of early marriage on offending (Knight, Osborn, and West, 1977). Marriage has often been invoked as the most effective treatment for male offending. In testing this, convictions and self-reports of offending at 18 were compared with convictions and self-reports at 21, according to whether the men did or did not marry between ages 18 and 21. No effect of marriage could be detected. The married and unmarried men decreased their offending between 18 and 21 at an approximately equal rate. However, later research on marriage up to age 24 suggests that the effects of marriage may depend to some extent on the characteristics of the wife. It seemed that men who married delinquent wives tended to get worse, while those who married non-delinquent wives tended to improve (West, 1982).

All these studies essentially used before-and-after measures of offending to evaluate the impact of events that occurred in between. Analyses based on more frequent measures would be more convincing because it would then be easier to pinpoint the exact timings of increases or decreases in offending and relate them to the time of occurrence of the events of interest. More analyses of this kind, making more use of the longitudinal nature of the data, should be carried out.

Implications for Criminological Theories

Ideally, there should be a relation between theory and research. Research should be used to generate theories, and theories should be used to guide research. However, many longitudinal researchers have not been particularly concerned with either generating or testing theories. There has been an emphasis on description rather than explanation. For example, the conclusion of Robins and Ratcliff (1980, p. 248) that "there exists a single syndrome made up of a broad variety of antisocial behaviors arising in childhood and continuing into adult-hood" is essentially an attempt to describe the phenomenon of continuity. Some researchers may have felt that it was premature to design research to test theories until some of the basic facts about the development and termination of delinquent behavior had been established. Certainly, some of the most influential theories in the history of criminology (e.g., Cohen, 1955) seem to be complex edifices not built on any secure foundation of empirical research, and it is questionable whether major resources should be devoted to testing such theories.

Existing longitudinal projects are useful in generating theories that can subsequently be tested, and longitudinal researchers should have attempted more of this kind of activity. The results of major longitudinal surveys pose a number of challenges to criminological theories. For example, why is there continuity in deviant behavior from childhood to adulthood? Why is deviant behavior versatile rather than specialized? Why does prevalence peak around ages 15 to 18? Why are those who start offending at the earliest ages the most persistent and frequent offenders? Why does the probability of offending increase with each successive offense? Why are parental child-rearing techniques, family criminality, the child's troublesome behavior, and the child's poor educational attainment the best predictors of the onset of offending? Why is so much offending concentrated in a small deviant minority, and why do convicted parents tend to have delinquent children? No doubt other questions could be proposed when we have a better understanding of what influences the rate of offending, the duration and termination of criminal careers, the types of offenses committed, and of events that can change the course of development of criminal careers.

In theory generation, there is often a choice between attempting to explain isolated results and proposing an all-embracing theory designed to explain everything. As an example of trying to explain isolated results, consider the finding that the probability of a subsequent arrest increases after each successive arrest. Blumstein *et al.* (1985) proposed a differential dropping out process to explain this, with the offenders containing successively more of the persisters as opposed to the desisters. An alternative theory is that some aspect of the official processing makes people more likely to commit crimes or to be arrested for them in the future, as Farrington (1977) found. Still another possibility is that people learn to offend as a result of the rewards and punishments experienced. A larger theory could be built up from these kinds of hypotheses proposed to explain isolated results.

As an example of a more comprehensive theory generated to explain the results of a longitudinal research project, the proposals of Farrington (1986c) will be described. He put forward an explanation inspired by aspects of five major theories: Cohen's (1955) delinquent subculture theory, Cloward and Ohlin's (1960) strain theory, Trasler's (1962) social learning theory, Hirschi's (1969) social control theory, and Sutherland and Cressey's (1974) differential association theory. Farrington's theory was intended to explain the most common varieties of male delinquency (crimes of dishonesty such as thefts and burglaries). He suggested that delinquent acts were the end product of a four stage process:

1. In the first stage, motivation arose. It was suggested that the main desires that ultimately produced delinquent acts were desires for material goods, status among intimates, and excitement. These desires may be culturally induced in general or may be a response to a specific situation (e.g., a desire for excitement arising from a feeling of boredom). It may be that the desire for excitement is greater among children from poorer families because excitement is more highly valued by lower-class people than by middle-class people because poorer children lead more boring lives or because poorer children are less able to postpone immediate gratification in favor of long-term goals (which may be linked to the emphasis in lower-class culture on the concrete and present as opposed to the abstract and future).

2. In the second stage, a legal or illegal method of satisfying the desire was chosen. It was suggested that some people (e.g., children from poorer families) were less able to satisfy their desires for material goods, excitement, and social status by legal or socially approved methods, and so they tended to choose illegal or socially disapproved methods. The relative inability of poorer children to achieve goals by legitimate methods may be partly because they tended to fail in school and hence tended to have erratic, low-status employment histories. School failure in turn was often a consequence of the unstimulating intellectual environment that lower-class parents tended to provide for their children and the lack of emphasis on abstract concepts.

3. In the third stage, a motivation to commit a delinquent act was magnified or opposed by internalized beliefs and attitudes about law-breaking, which had been built up in a learning process as a result of a history of rewards and punishments. The belief that delinquency was wrong, or a "strong conscience," tended to be built up if parents were in favor of legal norms, if they exercised close supervision over their children, and if they punished socially disapproved behavior using love-oriented discipline. The belief that delinquency was legitimate, and anti-establishment attitudes generally, tended to be built up if children had been exposed to attitudes and behavior favoring delinquency, especially by members of their family and their friends.

4. The fourth stage was a decision process in a particular situation and was affected by immediate situational factors. If any resulting motivation to commit a delinquent act survived the third stage, whether the tendency became the

actuality, in any given situation, depended on the costs, benefits, and probabilities of the possible outcomes (e.g., the material that could be stolen, peer approval, being caught by the police). In general, people were hedonistic and made rational decisions.

Applying this theory to the results obtained in the London longitudinal project, children from poorer families could have been especially likely to commit delinquent acts because they were unable to achieve their goals legally (partly because they tended to fail in school) and possibly because they valued some goals (e.g., excitement) especially highly. Children who received parental mishandling could have been especially likely to commit delinquent acts because they failed to build up internal controls over socially disapproved behavior, while children from criminal families and those with delinquent friends tended to build up anti-establishment attitudes and the belief that delinquency was justifiable. The whole process could have been self-perpetuating in that early school failure led to truancy (or truancy led to school failure) and to a lack of educational qualifications, which in turn led to low-status jobs and periods of unemployment, all of which made it even harder to achieve goals legitimately. Similarly, delinquent acts themselves could have causal effects because they could lead to official processing and hence to anti-establishment attitudes, delinquent friends, and unstable job histories.

Delinquency may peak between ages 14 and 20 because boys (especially lower-class school failures) had high desires for excitement, material goods, and status between these ages, little chance of achieving these desires legally, and little to lose (since legal penalties were lenient and their intimates—male peers—approved of delinquency). In contrast, after age 20, desires became attenuated or more realistic, there was more possibility of achieving these more limited goals legally, and the costs of delinquency were greater (since legal penalties were harsher and their intimates—wives or girlfriends—disapproved of delinquency).

This theory clearly needs more careful specification and testing. However, it does attempt to address some of the major results of existing longitudinal research in a way that other theories do not. Longitudinal surveys are especially useful in testing theories that emphasize stages of development or causal chains.

The most important recent attempt to test an all-embracing theory in a longitudinal project can be found in the work of Elliott, Huizinga, and Ageton (1985). They attempted to integrate strain, control, and social learning theories. One of their key ideas was that delinquency resulted from differential bonding to conventional and deviant groups. There were three alternative paths to delinquency. The strain theory path occurred when conventional bonding (produced by effective early childhood socialization) was attenuated by poor school performance and limited opportunities for achieving goals. Crime acted as an alternative method of achieving material success. The control theory path occurred when childhood socialization was ineffective, producing weak internal and external controls over delinquency. Essentially, strain theory was explaining why pressures toward deviance arose, while control theory explained why these pressures were not kept in check. The third, social learning, path occurred when delinquency was reinforced by an individual's interpersonal network. In the socialization process, conventional or deviant behavior could be reinforced, and the primary reinforcer for deviant behavior was the peer group. It followed that delinquency was most serious when strain, weak conventional bonding, and strong bonding to deviant groups occurred together.

Elliott *et al.* tested these ideas using measures of strain (family and school aspirations), conventional bonding (family and school involvement), and deviant bonding (involvement with delinquent peers, deviant attitudes). They carried out causal modeling analyses to investigate how far measures taken in 1976 and 1977 could predict self-reported delinquency in 1977 and how far measures taken in 1977 and 1978 could predict self-reported delinquency in 1978. The best predictor of self-reported delinquency was involvement with delinquent peers. In fact, only prior delinquency and involvement with delinquent peers had direct effects on delinquency in a path analysis. They concluded (p. 138) that "the only measure having a direct effect on delinquency and drug use was bonding to deviant peers, and the effects of strain and conventional bonding were almost totally indirect, mediated by the level of bonding to deviant peers."

There are a number of problems with this attempt to test an all-embracing theory in a longitudinal project. Most importantly, the analyses carried out by Elliott *et al.* are essentially correlational and have much in common with those used in cross-sectional surveys such as by Johnson (1979). These analyses cannot unambiguously demonstrate causal relationships. In particular, even if a measure of involvement with delinquent peers at one time predicts self-reported delinquency at a later time independent of some other possible predictor variables, this does not show that involvement with delinquent peers causes (or even precedes) delinquency. This relationship could merely reflect the facts that delinquency occurs in groups and that there is continuity in behavior. Also, as in any other essentially correlational study, the relationship could have been produced by other, unmeasured variables.

The research of Elliott *et al.* is clearly innovative and important. However, their results would be more compelling if they had carried out more clearly longitudinal analyses. For example, with even three data points, it would be possible to investigate if changes in involvement with delinquent peers between the first and the second were followed by changes in delinquency between the second and the third. It would also be possible to establish if these relationships held after controlling for other variables, and also to investigate other threats to internal validity as described by Cook and Campbell (1979). Basically, in testing theories or hypotheses derived from theories, what is needed is experimental or quasi-experimental research. Correlational analyses can never be convincing. This argument will be discussed in greater detail in Chapter 3.

Secondary Analyses

The data collected by longitudinal researchers has proved to be a useful resource for secondary analyses by other researchers. This is especially true of the influential project by Wolfgang *et al.* (1972). The reanalyses carried out by Blumstein and Moitra (1980) and Barnett and Lofaso (1985) have already been discussed. Two other examples of reanalyses of the Wolfgang *et al.* data were carried out by Clarke (1974, 1975). These are interesting examples of the use of longitudinal data to investigate important policy issues that the original researchers had not been concerned with. Clarke's 1974 study was concerned with the effectiveness of incapacitation as a penal aim in preventing offending. He concluded that each incarceration, lasting on average 9 months and costing an average $1,100, prevented only one index offense. His 1975 study was concerned with the effect of decriminalizing status offenses. It had been argued that this would have little effect on the cumulative prevalence of juvenile court processing because most status offenders also committed criminal offenses. However, in the Wolfgang *et al.* data, Clarke found that status offenders were not likely to recidivate and that most boys who committed criminal acts did not begin by committing status offenses. Therefore, there were important differences between status and criminal offenders.

Jensen (1976) also reanalyzed the Wolfgang *et al.* data, concluding (in opposition to the original authors) that achievement was more strongly related to delinquency than was race or social class. As other examples of reanalyses of a longitudinal survey, Wiatrowski, Griswold, and Roberts (1981) used the *Youth in Transition* data of Bachman *et al.* (1978) to test a social control theory of delinquency, and Rankin and Wells (1985) used the same data to study escalation from status to delinquent offenses with age.

In view of the costliness and difficulty of longitudinal research, it is clearly desirable that data collected should be made available in archives for secondary analyses. This can help to enhance the value, and justify the cost, of longitudinal projects. It is also desirable that projects should collect data on a wide variety of topics. The marginal costs of extra data collection may not be very high, but the benefits—in terms of usefulness to a variety of researchers—may be very great. In particular, longitudinal projects on offending should also collect data on other deviant acts, including drunkenness, drug use, sexual promiscuity, and psychiatric conditions. Similarly, it would be desirable for longitudinal projects on these other topics to collect information also about offending.

Limitations of Major Longitudinal Studies

The most important limitation of existing longitudinal studies is the lack of attention to impact questions. We have learned a great deal about the natural history of criminal careers but little about the effects of specific events on the course of development of these careers. From the point of view of explanation, prevention, and treatment, more experimental and quasi-experimental research is needed within longitudinal studies.

Other limitations of existing longitudinal studies have been alluded to already in this chapter. In particular, the infrequency of data collection has often made it difficult to pinpoint causal order, thus failing to utilize one of the greatest possible advantages of longitudinal surveys. Also, data has often been collected from a very limited range of sources, making it hard to disentangle true relationships between important theoretical constructs from artifactual ones reflecting common response biases. Also, as pointed out in the section "Desirable Features of Longitudinal Surveys," data collection from a variety of different sources helps to establish the reliability and validity of measures.

A major problem with existing surveys based on only one cohort is the difficulty of ascribing changes to aging, period, or cohort effects. This is more feasible in multiple cohort studies such as that of Shannon (1981), but not a great deal of separation of effects has been attempted. In the future, more multiple cohort longitudinal surveys are needed, and more attention should be paid to the problem of separating effects.

Existing longitudinal surveys have paid little attention to the possibility of reactive or testing effects. As already mentioned ("Uses and Advantages of Longitudinal Studies"), when these have been investigated, they have been found to be small. However, if data are collected more frequently, it will become more necessary to estimate the effects on subjects of being studied over a period. Also, existing surveys have paid little attention to regression effects. In general, subjects with high scores at one time will tend to regress toward the mean at a later time because of the random error component in all scores. It is necessary to distinguish real changes in scores from regression effects, and this is one of the aims of quasi-experimental analyses.

There are a number of practical problems that all longitudinal surveys have faced and that have caused difficulties (see also Farrington, 1979c). A major one is to obtain a long-term guarantee of funding. Most long-term surveys have not had such a guarantee, making it difficult for them to plan ahead. Long-term planning is necessary in order to get the fullest possible benefits from longitudinal research. Of course, with the best of planning, uncontrollable events can occur and can spoil the design of a project. For example, in the Wolfgang *et al.* (1972) survey, many of the records were destroyed in a fire, making it impossible to follow up the whole cohort beyond age 18. As far as possible, future projects should plan for such eventualities by keeping several copies of key data (such as names and dates of birth, which can be linked to computerized information).

Of course, one of the reasons why names and dates of birth are not kept in a machine-readable form is because of restrictions imposed by ethics committees. There is often a conflict between what is ideal for researchers and the protection of the rights of individuals, and this can limit the value of data collected. For example, the requirement that subjects sign informed consent forms clearly reduces the rate of participation in any survey, and it seems likely that the least cooperative persons tend to be the most deviant and hence the most interesting to criminological researchers. Even nonreactive research can be limited by the requirements of informed consent. For example, Janson (1981, p. 98) reported that the 1974 Data Act in Sweden "virtually brings to an end the large-scale use of registers and files for research purposes" because it was held that a person's records could not be searched unless that person had given permission. Fortunately, this requirement has not been maintained by the Swedish authorities. However, it may be that longitudinal surveys are more feasible in some places than in others.

Attrition can occur in longitudinal surveys for a variety of reasons other than informed consent requirements. Subjects can be lost through death, emigration, unknown addresses, and refusals to be interviewed. Locating subjects seems to be especially a problem in the United States. For example, in the Wolfgang (1974) survey, only 58% of the target sample of 974 could be interviewed at age 26. Many could not be located, despite three years of diligent searching, using the Selective Service address file, motor vehicle registrations, post office assistance, and other agencies. Fortunately, longitudinal surveys often have information about missing subjects and so can estimate the maximum error caused by attrition. However, it is desirable to minimize attrition as far as possible by devising in advance ways to have regular contact with the subjects and by planning strategies to locate them.

Many longitudinal surveys are limited by retrospective data collection, short follow-up periods, and small, unrepresentative, local samples. However, this is less true of the major projects reviewed in this chapter because of the method of selection specified in the section "Major Prospective Longitudinal Surveys." Longitudinal surveys have also been limited by the particular time period which they have covered. Multiple cohorts are desirable to facilitate generalization over time. A problem that longer-term surveys have to face is how to allow for inevitable changes in instrumentation, methodology, theories, and topics of interest over time. Existing surveys have paid insufficient attention to this problem, partly because their ability to plan ahead was limited.

One of the aims of cataloging some of the limitations and problems of existing major studies is in the hope that they can be overcome in the future. The surveys proposed in Chapter 8 are designed with both the contributions and the limitations of existing longitudinal studies in mind.

Conclusions

Existing longitudinal surveys have advanced our knowledge about criminal careers in particular. They have provided information about rates of participation in offending at different ages and have shown that cumulative arrest rates are much higher than previously thought. They have shown the extent of continuity in offending and in other deviant activities from childhood to adulthood and the fact that offending is versatile rather than specialized. They have demonstrated that participation in offending peaks around age 15 to 18 and that the early arrested people have the longest careers and the highest total number of offenses. They have also shown that criminal parents tend to have delinquent children and that the best predictors of the onset of offending are parental child-rearing techniques, the child's poor educational achievement, and the child's troublesome behavior. Finally, they have pointed to the concentration of offending in a small deviant minority of high-rate offenders who can be predicted at an early age by such factors as poor school behavior, economic deprivation, convicted parents, low intelligence, and poor parental child-rearing behavior.

While describing the achievements of major longitudinal studies, this chapter has also drawn attention to their limitations. More research is needed that focuses on the impact of specific events—especially the reactions of the criminal justice system—on the course of development of criminal careers. Similarly, more experimental and quasi-experimental longitudinal studies are needed and more attempts to generate and test theories. More prospective studies, with more frequent data collection and obtaining data from a wider variety of sources, are also required. In addition, more surveys using multiple cohorts are desirable. We now turn to Chapter 3, which reviews what we have learned from experimental studies, and their limitations.

3
What Have We Learned From Major Experimental Studies?

Introduction

What Is an Experiment?

The word "experiment" is often used loosely to refer to any innovative change whose effects are uncertain. Technically, however, it refers to a systematic attempt to test a causal hypothesis about the effect of variations in one factor (the independent variable) on another (the dependent variable). The technical meaning will be used here. The defining feature of an experiment lies in the control of the independent variable by the experimenter.

It is easiest to explain the essential characteristics of an experiment by discussing a specific example. The Cambridge–Somerville Youth Study is one of the most famous criminological experiments of all time. It was designed to investigate whether delinquency could be prevented by providing friendly help, counseling, and desirable role models at an early age to boys who were thought to be at risk of becoming delinquents.

In Massachusetts in the 1930s, 650 boys were rated on delinquency potential by teachers and social agency representatives. They were divided into 325 pairs, with the members of each pair matched on delinquency potential and on certain other factors (age, intelligence, physical health, home, and neighborhood characteristics). One member of each pair was then chosen at random, by the toss of a coin, to receive the special help (lasting on average five years), while the other was left to the usual resources of the community. All the boys were then followed up to see whether the special help was effective in preventing delinquency. Unfortunately, it was not. Both short-term (Powers and Witmer, 1951) and long-term (McCord, 1978) follow-ups showed that the treated boys were at least as delinquent and criminal as the controls.

This study, which will be discussed further in the section "Community Prevention," shows the essential features of an experiment. The independent variable was the treatment—special help or not. The dependent variable was delinquent or criminal behavior. In investigating the effect of special help on delinquent behavior, the independent variable was under the control of the experimenter, since the experimenter determined who received the special help.

Furthermore, the fact that the boys were randomly assigned to treated and control groups meant that those in one group were equivalent, within the limits of statistical fluctuation, to those in the other. Many factors might influence delinquency, and the purpose of the randomization was to equate the groups on factors extraneous to the experiment. This control of extraneous variables by randomization made it possible to disentangle the effects of the treatment from the effects of any other influences on delinquency. If the treated group had proved to be less delinquent than the controls, it could have been concluded with confidence that in some way the treatment had succeeded in preventing delinquency. Equally, since the treated and control groups proved to be equivalent on delinquency, it could be concluded that providing friendly help, counseling, and desirable role models at an early age was ineffective in preventing delinquency.

Advantages of Randomized Experiments

Randomized experiments can establish the effect of one factor on another more securely than any other method because of the control of independent and extraneous variables. The more usual correlational research seen in criminology always leads to ambiguities in interpretation. For example, if a retrospective study had been carried out showing that counseled boys were less delinquent than other boys, it would be impossible to know whether the difference was caused by the counseling or whether it reflected one of the other uncontrolled differences between the groups. Only a randomized experiment can control all extraneous variables, and then only if a reasonably large number of people (at least 50) are assigned to each condition.

The control of extraneous variables by randomization is similar to the control of extraneous variables in the physical sciences by holding physical conditions (e.g., temperature, pressure) constant. Randomization ensures that the average unit in one treatment group is approximately equivalent to the average unit in another before the treatment is applied. Holding physical conditions constant ensures a more exact equivalence of experimental units, but the theory of experimental control is the same in both cases.

A more common method used to control extraneous variables is matching. This can be done prospectively in an experiment, for example, by matching people in different conditions on a small number of variables that are likely to be related to the dependent measure (e.g., age, sex, race, number of previous convictions, type of current offense). Alternatively, persons subjected to different treatments could be matched retrospectively. Whatever method is used, the major problem with matching is that it cannot ensure equivalence on all extraneous variables—only on a subset. It could always be argued that differences in outcome reflected differences in unmatched extraneous variables rather than differences in treatments.

Another way of achieving equivalent groups is to give all treatments to the same people in a random order, and this is the method favored in behavior modification research (see, e.g., Farrington, 1979a). However, in these "within-subjects" designs, people who receive one treatment second are not necessarily equivalent to those who receive the other treatment second because of the different effects of the treatments received first. Therefore, the emphasis here will be on "between-subjects" designs, in which each person receives only one of the treatments.

What Have We Learned?

This chapter will review the major randomized experiments that have been carried out on the prevention and treatment of crime and delinquency, including research on community treatment, institutional treatment, the police, and the courts. "Prevention" refers to attempts to reduce offending by measures taken before crimes occur, while "treatment" refers to attempts to reduce offending by measures taken after crimes occur. Most research in criminology has been nonexperimental or correlational in nature, leading to ambiguities in interpretation and controversial disagreements. A good example of this is the "suppression effect" of Murray and Cox (1979). They found that the arrest rate of chronic male offenders in Chicago declined by about two-thirds after they had served an average 11-month institutional sentence, while the arrest rate of comparable offenders dealt with in the community (by the "Unified Delinquency Intervention Services") declined less.

The two key questions are: Did the institutional program cause a reduction in crime? Was it more effective in this respect than the community program? Maltz, Gordon, McDowall, and McCleary (1980) argued that the decline after institutionalization could reflect a selection–regression artefact. In other words, if offending rates are fluctuating around some average value, institutionalization will tend to occur after an abnormally high rate of offending and the normal variation will then cause an apparent decline after release. This decline would be especially noticeable when comparing a short period before institutionalization with a short period after, as Murray and Cox did in their major comparison. This issue could be resolved by following up for a much longer period before and after the institutional treatment. The fluctuations, and the effect of the treatment, would then be more apparent (as would more general aging effects).

The second problem, commonly found in nonexperimental research, is whether the institutional and community groups were truly equivalent in all respects before the treatment. If not, it is difficult to disentangle the effects of the treatments from the effects of preexisting differences. J. Q. Wilson (1980) pointed out that because the youths in the community programs were specially selected, they were probably less dangerous and more amenable than the institutional youths. In light of this argument, it is surprising that the arrest rate of the community youths declined less. This result would have been more compelling if both groups (drawn perhaps from a high-risk population) had been followed up in a longitudinal survey and then randomly assigned to the institutional or community treatment. The random assignment would have achieved truly equivalent groups. Without it, there is always the suspicion that the institutional youths, although probably more dangerous and violent, were in fact less persistent to start with than the community youths.

Because of the methodological superiority of studies based on experiments, it is not surprising that the small number that have been carried out have attracted a great deal of attention and have proved especially influential. In particular, the major conclusion about the ineffectiveness of correctional treatments by Martinson (1974) and Sechrest, White, and Brown (1979), which has been one of the most important general findings of the last 20 years, was largely based on experimental research. There is little doubt that this finding would not have achieved such widespread acceptance if it had not been based on this method. However, we also hope to show in this chapter that some experiments lead to optimism about the effectiveness of prevention and treatment. The optimistic results require further testing by the most convincing method—the longitudinal-experimental technique (see Chapter 8). We also hope to show that, while randomized experiments are not common in criminology, a surprising number have been carried out successfully (see also Farringon, 1983c).

Our emphasis is on experiments on real-life problems carried out in real-life settings. There are considerable problems of generalization with more artificial experiments, such as the "simulated prison" study of Haney, Banks, and Zimbardo (1973). Again, because of the need for reasonably large numbers in order to achieve the benefits of randomization, experiments involving less than about 50 subjects per condition will not be reviewed. However, experiments on larger units than persons (e.g., areas), which almost inevitably involve less than 50 per condition, will be reviewed later in the section "Experiments on Larger Units."

Experiments inevitably require a prospective longitudinal design. The dependent variable is usually measured only after the manipulation of the independent variable. However, the dependent variable could be measured both before and after, as in a pretest–posttest design. An advantage of pretest measurement is that it can help to verify that the random assignment was successful in producing equivalent groups. Furthermore, pretest measurement can provide valuable information about the state of affairs on which the manipulation is intended to have an impact and, hence, can increase the likelihood of discovering interactions between types of persons and types of treatments.

Perhaps the major reason why the experimental method is not common in criminology is because of the ethical, legal, and practical problems involved. (Some of these will be discussed in Chapter 8.) When experimentation is not feasible, the next best method of testing a causal hypothesis is to take advantage of a naturally occurring event and analyze its effects as if it had been manipulated experimentally. Some examples of this "quasi-experimental" research will be reviewed in the section "Quasi-Experiments."

Experiments and Scientific Progress

It is unlikely that any single experiment in criminology could be a crucial test of a causal hypothesis because of differing operational definitions of theoretical constructs and boundary conditions. For example, we should not conclude from the Cambridge–Somerville study alone that counseling is ineffective in preventing delinquency, but that counseling as provided in this project is ineffective. It is possible that other definitions of counseling would be effective in preventing other definitions of delinquency or even that this kind of counseling would have prevented this kind of delinquency with other kinds of persons or in other kinds of places. [However, the failure of several other experiments to affect delinquency or crime using counseling (see below) leads us to have little confidence in counseling as a method of prevention or treatment.]

Ideally, each experiment should be one link in a chain of cumulative knowedge guided by theory. In the classic model of scientific progress, a series of testable causal hypotheses is derived from each theory. If each hypothesis is tested in an experiment, the pattern of results can be compared to the pattern of theoretical predictions. On the basis of this comparison, and taking into account other considerations such as the complexity of a theory, it is possible to conclude that one theory is preferable to another.

At the present time, criminology lags far behind the physical sciences: well-developed, explicitly specified, falsifiable theories are rare in criminology. This is why many criminological problems require a two-stage approach. In the first stage, hypotheses, ideas, or theories are generated, while in the second stage these are tested empirically. There are many ways of generating hypotheses, including armchair reflection, scrutiny of relevant literature, participant or non-participant observation of the phenomenon, structured or unstructured interviews, and searches of relevant records. Longitudinal research is also useful for this purpose. However, except for hypotheses that require this method (such as those referring to the natural history of criminal careers), it is probably too expensive a resource to use in generating hypotheses. The experimental method is the best way of testing hypotheses. Unfortunately, many criminologists seem to value generating hypotheses more than testing them, and this is one of the reasons why experimentation is not common. The most influential of present-day criminological theories (e.g., Elliott et al., 1985; Hirschi, 1969) were generated and tested in research projects that are essentially nonexperimental.

Hypotheses tested in experiments are usually isolated ideas rather than part of a program of systematic testing of a larger theory. There is little attempt to see how far these hypotheses are true over different operational definitions of independent and dependent variables or different boundary conditions. In order to establish the causes of crime and to determine the best methods of preventing and treating it, criminology needs to move farther along the road of scientific progress. Randomized experiments represent a significant step in the right direction.

Prevention Experiments

Preschool Prevention

One of the most interesting attempts to prevent delinquency was the Perry preschool project carried out in Michigan by Schweinhart and Weikart (1980).

This was essentially a "Head Start" program targeted on disadvantaged black children who were allocated (approximately at random) to experimental and control groups. The experimental children attended a daily preschool program, backed up by weekly home visits, usually lasting two years (covering ages 3 and 4). The aim of the program was to provide intellectual stimulation, to increase cognitive abilities, and to increase later school achievement.

More than 120 children in the two groups were followed up to age 15 by means of teacher ratings, parent and youth interviews, and school records. As demonstrated in several other Head Start projects, the experimental group showed short-lived gains in intelligence (being 12 points ahead of the control group at ages 4 and 5, 5 points ahead at age 7, but no different at age 14). However, the experimental group was significantly better in elementary school motivation, school achievement at 14, teacher ratings of classroom behavior at 6 to 9, self-reports of classroom behavior at 15, *and* on self-reported offending at 15. Furthermore, a later follow-up of this sample by Berrueta-Clement, Schweinhart, Barnett, Epstein, and Weikart (1984) showed that, at age 19, the experimental group was more likely to be employed, more likely to have graduated from high school, more likely to have received college or vocational training, and less likely to have been arrested or charged (31% as opposed to 51% of the control group).

These results suggest that a preschool intellectual enrichment program can lead to increased school success and ultimately to decreased delinquency and crime. We have known for a long time that school success and delinquency are negatively correlated, so this project confirms the expectation that changes in school success will be followed by changes in delinquency.

The findings in the Perry study are admittedly based on small numbers. However, they become more compelling when viewed in the context of the other projects followed up by the Consortium for Longitudinal Studies (1983). Every well-designed experimental Head Start preschool early intervention project aiming to enhance children's cognitive development and carried out in the 1960s was invited to join the Consortium to collect comparable follow-up data in 1976 and 1980. In general, the follow-up studies showed that the early intervention programs had beneficial effects on school success in the long term, especially in increasing the rate of high school graduation and in decreasing the rate of special education placements. The Perry project was the only one to include data on delinquency and crime, but the consistency of results in all 11 projects in showing increases in school success suggests that the delinquency results might be replicable.

School Prevention

The two most important school experiments on delinquency prevention were carried out by Meyer, Borgatta, and Jones (1965) and Reckless and Dinitz (1972). Meyer *et al.* carried out their research in a vocational high school in New York City. Nearly 400 girls thought to have potential behavior problems were randomly assigned either to an experimental group, which received case work or group counseling from school social workers, or to a control group. A three year follow-up revealed no significant differences between the groups in suspensions or discharges from school, truancy, teachers' ratings of conduct, pregnancies out of wedlock, or court appearances. Reasonably, Meyer *et al.* concluded that the social work intervention had no effect on delinquency.

Reckless and Dinitz were interested in testing the theory that improvements in self-concept, achieved in internalizing more appropriate role models, would lead to decreases in delinquency. In Columbus, Ohio, teachers in 44 elementary schools were asked to rate all sixth-grade boys according to their likelihood of becoming delinquent. The researchers were then able to assign over 1,000 of the most vulnerable boys at random to either experimental or regular seventh-grade classes. The experimental classes were staffed by project teachers who aimed to present appropriate role model materials and who also concentrated on remedial reading.

The results of the experiment showed that the special classes had little effect on either delinquency or factors known to be related to delinquency. The experimental and control boys were not significantly different in school performance up to the tenth grade, in truancy, or in dropping out of school. The prevalence of police contacts during the one-year program was 12% for the experimental group and 11% for the control group, while the prevalence of police contacts during the following three years was 38% and 36%, respectively. Furthermore, follow-up interviews two years after the seventh grade showed that the experimental and control groups were not significantly different in self-reports of offending. They were also no different on a self-concept inventory, suggesting that the special classes had not been effective in improving the self-concept. Nonetheless, 97% of the experimental boys said that they were glad that they had had the different kind of seventh-grade class.

These experiments have advanced our knowledge by showing that two methods of intervention in school—social work treatment and special classes designed to improve the self-concept—had no effect on delinquency. The Reckless and Dinitz experiment is especially impressive in view of the large numbers of children involved and the use of both official and self-report measures of offending. It is important to note that experiments with negative results, if they are competently carried out, can advance our knowledge about crime just as much as those with more positive findings (see also Chapter 4).

Community Prevention

The most important community prevention experiment—the Cambridge-Somerville study—has already been described briefly in the section "What Is an Experiment?" The experimental boys in this study received an average of five years of regular friendly attention from counselors, while the control boys were left to the usual resources of the community. Unfortunately, the 30-year follow-up by McCord (1978) showed that the treatment had been ineffectual. About a quarter of both groups were known to have committed crimes as juveniles, while about two-thirds of both groups had been convicted as adults.

Worse than this, what differences there were in this study showed that the control group had a more satisfactory life. Significantly more of the experimental group committed two or more crimes, became alcoholics, developed mental illness, suffered from stress-related diseases, and died at an early age. Nevertheless, two-thirds of the experimental group said that the program had been helpful to them, usually by providing interesting activities to keep them out of trouble or by teaching them how to get along with others.

In trying to explain the failure of the community program, McCord speculated that the intervention might have created a dependency on outside assistance, which in turn led to resentment when the assistance was withdrawn. Alternatively, the treatment program might have generated high expectations that subsequently led to feelings of deprivation when the expectations were not met. Another possibility was that the treated group may have justified the treatment they received by perceiving themselves as being in need of welfare help. Whatever the true reason, McCord drew the important conclusion that programs could end up damaging the persons they were intended to help. This emphasizes the need for careful experimental evaluations of such programs.

Another interesting community prevention experiment was carried out in Hawaii by Fo and O'Donnell (1974, 1975). More than 500 youths referred for behavior or academic problems were randomly assigned either to have adult "buddies" or not. The buddies met regularly with the youths in their natural environment and tried to influence them to engage in socially approved behavior, giving priority to school attendance. The buddies tried to influence the youths using behavioral techniques (especially contingency management). The buddies earned points, which were exchangeable for money, for specific acts such as making weekly contact with youths, completing weekly assignments with them, or attending a training session.

Overall, the project had little effect on delinquency. Combining the one year of the project and a two-year follow-up period, 32% of the experimental group were arrested, in comparison with 28% of the controls (O'Donnell, Lydgate, and Fo, 1979). However, there seemed to be some interaction between types of persons and the treatment since the arrest rate was lower for the experimental group among those with offenses in the previous year and higher for the experimental group among those with no offenses in the previous year. Both of these effects were statistically weak. However, if they are taken seriously, it seems that this kind of behaviorally based community help may be beneficial to offenders but harmful to nonoffenders.

Perhaps the most interesting recent prevention experiment was carried out in St. Louis by Feldman et al. (1983). As mentioned in Chapter 2, delinquency is largely a group activity. If deviant peers facilitate offending, as is often argued (e.g., Elliott et al., 1985), it should be possible to reduce delinquency either by reducing exposure to deviant peers or by increasing exposure to prosocial peers. This was the theoretical basis for the St. Louis project.

Feldman *et al.* studied over 400 boys who were referred because of antisocial behavior and randomly assigned them to two kinds of activity groups, each comprising about 10–12 adolescents. The groups either consisted entirely of referred youths or consisted of one or two referred youths and about 10 nonreferred (prosocial) peers. Feldman *et al.* found that, on the basis of systematic observations, self-reports by the youths, and ratings by the group leaders, the antisocial behavior of the referred youths in mixed groups (with prosocial peers) decreased relative to that of the referred youths in unmixed groups. It is unfortunate that the number of referred youths in mixed groups was small. However, this result is in conformity with the attempt by Sarason (1978) to reduce delinquency in peer groups using prosocial models (see the section "Other Institutional Treatments"). It suggests that the peer group can have an important role in producing, maintaining, and reducing delinquency.

Deterrent or Moral Appeals

Schwartz and Orleans (1967) were interested in investigating whether the threat of punishment was effective in deterring people from committing crimes. The crime they studied was income tax evasion. Nearly 300 taxpayers drawn from high-income areas were randomly assigned to three groups. Two of the groups were interviewed during the month before income tax returns had to be filed, in one case stressing the penalties for income tax evasion and in the other stressing moral reasons for tax compliance. The third group was not interviewed and served as a control. The Internal Revenue Service provided details of the taxes paid by all three groups for the year before and the year during which the experiment was carried out. Interestingly, Schwartz and Orleans discovered that the moral appeal led to a significant increase in the tax paid, whereas the sanction threat had no effect.

Community Treatment Experiments

Diversion from the Juvenile Court

As will be pointed out in Chapter 6, programs designed to divert juveniles from the juvenile court proliferated during the 1970s, partly based on the belief that the court had undesirable stigmatizing effects rather than desirable rehabilitative ones. A number of these diversion programs have been evaluated in controlled experiments.

The earliest and possibly most encouraging experiment was carried out by Baron, Feeney, and Thornton (1973). Instead of being handled by the regular intake unit, for four days a week (out of 7) Sacramento juvenile offenders were handled by a special diversion unit that relied on family crisis counseling.

Because the days of the week on which the diversion unit operated were rotated monthly (Baron and Feeney, 1976), this experiment involved an assignment process that was quite close to random. Especially for criminal offenders, but also for status offenders, the recidivism rates were lower for those who were dealt with by the diversion unit.

Another interesting diversion experiment was carried out in Costa Mesa and Huntington Beach, California, by Binder, Monahan, and Newkirk (1976). This was a comparison between a diversion program and no treatment rather than between a diversion program and the regular court intake unit. The program was based on behavioral principles and aimed to teach parents effective ways of giving rewards and imposing sanctions, to teach juveniles coping skills, to teach families effective methods of communication, and to provide volunteer adult models for long-term imitation and friendship (Binder and Newkirk, 1977). The published papers show that the diversion group had a lower recidivism rate during a one-year follow-up period than the controls, and interviews with the juveniles and their parents also showed that the diversion group was better behaved. However, a later unpublished report (Binder, 1978) indicates that these positive results were only obtained in one of the two cities (Costa Mesa).

Encouraging results were also reported in a diversion experiment by Quay and Love (1977), but these now seem a little more doubtful. In Florida, more than 550 children referred by the court and other social agencies were randomly assigned either to a diversion program or to a control group, which was dealt with by other means available to the juvenile justice system. The diversion program consisted of vocational and personal counseling and academic education. Significantly fewer of the diverted juveniles were rearrested after the program (32% as opposed to 45% of the controls).

Unfortunately, Mrad (1979) then pointed out that these results could reflect the differential follow-up periods and the fact that arrests while the juveniles were in the diversion program were not counted. He showed that, when days in the program were added to the follow-up period afterward, the diverted group had an average rearrest rate of 40% in an average 400 days, while the control group had an average rearrest rate of 45% in an average 450 days. This suggested that the diversion program had been ineffective. In reply, Quay and Love (1979) argued that there was a significant difference between the groups even if the follow-up period was standardized at 300 days, so it is possible that this counseling-based diversion program had some effect on juvenile offending.

Byles and Maurice (1979) published an experimental evaluation of a diversion program in Hamilton, Canada, based on crisis-oriented family therapy. Over 300 juveniles who were apprehended by the police for alleged offenses were randomly assigned either to the diversion program or to the regular youth bureau. A two-year follow-up showed that the two groups were not significantly different in recidivism rates, which were high in both cases (62% for the diverted juveniles and 55% for the controls).

An impressive diversion experiment was carried out by Severy and Whitaker (1982). They were able to compare a special community-based diversion program not only with more traditional processing through the juvenile court but also with no treatment at all (the juveniles merely being released with no further action). Again unlike other diversion experiments, this study was restricted to youths who had committed serious offenses, who would normally go to court. In Memphis, Tennessee, over 2,200 youths were randomly assigned to the three conditions, and the recidivism rates in a one-year follow-up period were remarkably similar in all cases. The major problem in interpreting these results is to know what the diversion program consisted of in practice, but it is particularly interesting that the juvenile court processing had the same effect on recidivism as no treatment at all.

The most ambitious experimental evaluation of diversion projects was completed in four cities by Dunford, Osgood, and Weichselbaum (1982). Youths arrested for delinquent acts were randomly assigned to receive diversion with services, diversion without services, or further penetration into the juvenile justice system. The most common types of services were counseling, recreational, employment, or educational. The results showed no difference between the three conditions in self-reported or official offending during a one-year follow-up period.

It is difficult to summarize these results because of the heterogeneity of the diversion programs. However, in general, the more traditional programs based on counseling did not seem to be very effective, as was the case with most other experiments on counseling quoted here. The most hopeful kind of diversion program is probably the behaviorally based one of Binder and his colleagues.

Probation Supervision

One of the earliest experiments on probation supervision was carried out by Venezia (1972) in California. Over 120 juveniles who were designated for unofficial probation (thereby avoiding a court appearance) were randomly assigned either to probation supervision or to be counseled and released. The two groups had similar recidivism rates during a six-month follow-up period. It is unfortunate that the numbers were rather small and the follow-up period rather short in this experiment, but the results do not increase our confidence in the effectiveness of probation supervision.

The effects of intensive as opposed to regular probation were studied in two experiments, one American and one English. In Detroit, Lichtman and Smock (1981) randomly assigned over 500 male adult offenders either to regular probation or to a special variety in which the probation officers had low caseloads and assistance from citizen volunteers. The experimental subjects had twice as much contact with their probation officers as the controls (2.4 as opposed to 1.3 contacts per month on average) but were no different in reconvictions during a two- to three-year follow-up period.

Very similar results were obtained in the English experiment by Folkard, Smith, and Smith (1976). Over 900 adults in four areas of England were randomly assigned either to regular probation or to a special intensive variety in which the officers had low caseloads and were relieved of other office duties. As in the American study, the experimental subjects had twice as much contact with their probation officers as the controls (3 as opposed to 1.5 contacts per month on average) but were no different in reconvictions during a two-year follow-up period.

In another English experiment, Berg (Berg, Consterdine, Hullin, McGuire, and Tyrer, 1978; Berg, Hullin, and McGuire, 1979) investigated the effectiveness of supervision for juvenile truancy cases. The supervision could be carried out either by probation officers or by social workers. About 100 children appearing before the Leeds juvenile court for truancy were randomly assigned either to supervision or to a repeated adjournment (continuance) procedure. A six-month follow-up period showed that those who were supervised had worse school attendance records and higher delinquency rates than the remainder.

Finally, Holden (1983) studied the effectiveness of different methods of dealing with drinking drivers in Memphis, Tennessee. Over 4,100 drinking drivers with no prior convictions for this offense were randomly assigned to either probation or no probation and to either an education and therapy program for drinkers or no such program. Holden found no difference between the various conditions in drunk driving rearrest rates during a two-year follow-up period, suggesting that neither probation nor the program was effective.

These well-designed experiments on probation supervision suggest that it has little or no effect on offending. In view of the minimal nature of most such supervision (usually consisting of one or two short meetings per month), this is not surprising. Supervision seemed notably ineffective in the Berg research on truants, and this may reflect the deterrent effect of the alternative (adjournment) procedure. The children who were adjourned were told by the Court that they would be sent to a residential institution for a few weeks if their school attendance did not improve. This happened less often to the children who were supervised because the supervisors (probation officers and social workers) did everything they could to avoid such placements. Deterrence, therefore, may be more effective than counseling.

Alternatives to Incarceration

Some of the best known, classic examples of criminological experiments—the California Community Treatment Program, the Provo and Silverlake experiments—involved comparisons between youths incarcerated and others selected at random to receive treatment in the community. In the Community Treatment Program, Sacramento and Stockton youths who would normally be sent to an institution for 8–10 months were instead (after 4 weeks in a reception center) given parole with relatively intensive supervision. Attempts were made to match the youths and their parole officers, who were specially selected and who had low caseloads. Each youth received differential treatment according to interpersonal maturity level (see Palmer, 1971), and the program could involve counseling, residence in a group home, school teaching, surveillance by parole officers, and detention in an institution.

Palmer (1974) reported the results of the project separately for the periods 1961–69 and 1969–74. In the earlier period, boys randomly assigned to the program had lower recidivism rates during a two-year follow-up period than those sent to an institution. There was no difference for girls. However, Lerman (1975) has cast doubt on the effectiveness of the program for boys, pointing out that the program and institution groups had equal rearrest rates but different probabilities of having their parole revoked after an arrest. (The recidivism measure was the parole revocation rate.) He concluded that the program had succeeded in changing the discretionary decision-making behavior of adult correctional officials but had not had an appreciable effect on the behavior of the youths.

In the later period of the project, there seemed to be a differential effect of the program according to prior characteristics of the offenders. Palmer (1978) reported that for "conflicted" males, those randomly assigned to the community program had lower monthly arrest rates (during their youth authority career and a four-year postdischarge period) than those who received residential treatment. However, for "power-oriented" males, the differences were insignificant or the arrest rates were higher in the community program. As in the experiment by Adams (1970; discussed in the section "Counseling and Group Therapy"), this shows that the effects of correctional treatment may not be the same for all types of offenders. J. Q. Wilson (1980) summarized these results by pointing out that the young, anxious, verbal, intelligent, neurotic (Yavin) offenders were the most amenable to treatment.

The Provo experiment (Empey and Erickson, 1972) was targeted on male repeat offenders in Utah. Offenders who were eligible for the program were given probation or incarceration by a judge and were then randomly assigned either to the judge's disposition or to the program. As designed, the experiment was intended to compare the community program with probation and with incarceration. Unfortunately, this plan broke down because of the judge's reluctance to institutionalize offenders. Therefore, the most valid comparisons in this experiment are between the community program and probation. Nevertheless, this experiment is included in this section because it was presented by the authors as one of the first attempts to establish and evaluate a community alternative to incarceration for serious offenders, and it is regarded as such by criminologists.

Boys in the community program lived at home and spent part of each day at the program center, where the emphasis was on guided group interaction and on work. If a boy failed to attend satisfactorily, he was taken back to court and sent to an institution. The results of this experiment showed that the community program was no more effective than regular probation in preventing reoffending. The report is particularly interesting in presenting before-and-after measures of offending. The number of recorded offenses in the four years before the experiment and in the four years after were very similar for the program and probation groups.

The rate of offending after was only about one-third of the rate before. However, this does not necessarily mean that both the program and probation had significant effects in reducing offending. As Maltz *et al.* (1980) pointed out in commenting on the similar "suppression" effect of Murray and Cox (1979), the results could be due to a selection–regression artefact (see earlier). In other words, if offending rates are fluctuating around some average value, it is likely that probation and incarceration will follow a higher than average rate of offending. Because of the fluctuation, these dispositions will then be followed by a lower than average rate. Perhaps more important, the Provo boys had an average age of 16½, and therefore may have been at their peak age of offending. The decline in recorded offending during the next four years could reflect known changes in offending with age.

The Silverlake experiment (Empey and Lubeck, 1971), carried out in Los Angeles, was a more successful comparison of institutional and community treatment. As in the Provo experiment, the subjects were male repeat offenders aged 15 to 17, and the community program was based on guided group interaction. However, unlike the Provo experiment, boys who would normally have been sent to an institution were randomly assigned either to the institution (which had a highly structured, regimented living environment) or to the community program. The results showed no significant difference in recidivism between the two treatments. As in the Provo experiment, the rate of recorded offending declined in both cases from the period before the intervention to the period after.

Another notable community treatment experiment was carried out in California by Lamb and Goertzel (1974). From a sample of offenders sentenced to the county jail, half were randomly assigned to a community rehabilitation center. Both groups were then followed up for six months in the community, and they did not differ significantly in the parole revocation rate. This rate was considerably higher in the community group (27% as opposed to 17%), but the small numbers (110 in total) precluded a significant difference.

Summarizing the results of this section, these experiments show that community treatment based on counseling or guided group interaction is no more or less effective in preventing recidivism than institutionalization, for all offenders. However, there may be differential effects for different types of offenders.

Institutional Treatment Experiments

Counseling and Group Therapy

One of the earliest experiments on individual counseling inside an institution was carried out in California by Adams (1970). About 1,600 institutionalized delinquents were randomly assigned either to a group that received counseling once or twice a week for an average of nine months or to a control group that did not receive such counseling. In addition, the offenders were classified as amenable to counseling or nonamenable. The first 100 releasees in each of the four possible categories (treated amenable, treated nonamenable, nontreated amenable, non-treated nonamenable) were followed up for about 33 months.

The results showed that, overall, counseling had little effect on recidivism. However, as in the experiment by Palmer (1978), there appeared to be an interesting interaction between the type of person and the type of treatment. The treated amenables had the lowest recidivism rate, while the treated nonamenables had the highest. A slight problem in this experiment is that the persons followed up (the first 100 releasees in each condition) had not been randomly assigned. The randomization ensured comparability of all treated and all control youths, but whether treated youths released first were comparable to control youths released first is less certain.

The most important study of group counseling in an institution was carried out in California by Kassebaum, Ward, and Wilner (1971) in which they were able to take advantage of the opening of a new prison with separate living units. (There are often problems in randomly assigning inmates to existing living units because the randomized inmates may be influenced by nonrandomized inmates who are already present. This problem was avoided in the Kassebaum *et al.* study.) Special categories of prisoners such as the psychotic, aged, homosexual, and young "management problems," were assigned to one living area, while all other prisoners were randomly assigned to living units elsewhere in the new prison.

The most important comparisons in the Kassebaum *et al.* study were between those who received large-group counseling, those who received small-group counseling, and controls who received no counseling. The group counseling involved meetings between staff and inmates about once or twice a week to talk over matters of concern, aiming to build up warm, supportive relationships between staff and inmates. There was also an attempt to develop something approaching a "therapeutic community" in the group counseling living units. However, a three-year follow-up showed no significant differences in recidivism between the conditions. If anything, those who received large-group counseling had the worst outcome, but then they had somewhat the worst prognosis to start with, according to Base Expectancy scores.

Major objections to this project were voiced by Quay (1977). He argued that this experiment was not a valid test of the efficacy of group counseling because the service was delivered by minimally trained and inexpert personnel. There was no attempt to match the treatment to the individual. He thought that group counseling as a "group setting necessary for clients to feel free to discuss with security their own and each others' feelings and attitudes toward the situation in which they find themselves" (p. 352) was never achieved. However, while this experiment may not have been a valid test of the ideal type of group counseling (as a theoretical construct), it may have been a valid test of the kind of group counseling more typically employed in prisons.

Other experiments on the efficacy of group counseling or the therapeutic community have been carried out in Canada by Annis (1979) and in England by Cornish and Clarke (1975) and Williams (1970, 1975). Annis randomly assigned 150 male prisoners with alcohol or drug problems either to receive two types of group therapy or to be in a control group. The group therapy was quite intensive, occupying seven hours a day for four days a week for eight weeks, but it had no effect on reconvictions during a one-year follow-up period.

Cornish and Clarke compared one living unit in a juvenile institution that operated as a therapeutic community with another living unit with a more traditional regime. The therapeutic regime was based on group meetings, aimed for decisions made jointly by staff and inmates, and was permissive to rebellious behavior, while the traditional regime emphasized discipline and hard work and used mainly individual counseling to deal with the boys' underlying problems. The staff were chosen to be sympathetic to the regime in which they were operating. From nearly 300 boys allocated to the institution, the therapeutic staff selected nearly 200 who they thought could benefit from their regime, and these were randomly assigned either to the therapeutic community or to the traditional living unit. However, a two-year follow-up showed no difference between the two conditions in reconviction rates, with about two-thirds reconvicted in both cases.

Williams compared three different English institutions for young male offenders, one employing a traditional regime (paternalistic control with an emphasis on self-discipline and hard work), the second emphasizing individual casework or counseling, and the third emphasizing group counseling. Offenders were randomly assigned to the institutions, and Williams waited until the institutions were full of randomly assigned offenders before beginning to collect data. The results of this experiment showed that offenders dealt with in the casework institution had significantly lower reconviction rates in a two-year follow-up period than those deal with in the other two institutions (51% as opposed to 63% in the other two). However, it is possible that the success of the casework institution was produced artefactually. This institution had the highest rate of transferring offenders to other institutions, and the transferred offenders (who were usually absconders) tended to have high reconviction rates.

To conclude, the experiments on individual and group counseling in institutions do not demonstrate clearly that these methods are superior to alternative treatment techniques in reducing recidivism, although again there may be differential effects for different types of offenders (see also Chapter 7).

Other Institutional Treatments

Experiments have been carried out to investigate the efficacy of a variety of other institutional treatment methods. Three of the most important of these were carried out in California by Jesness (1971a, 1971b, 1975). The Preston typology study (Jesness, 1971b) was an elaborate attempt to match the treaters and the treatment to the treated youths. There were six experimental living units and five control ones, and about 100 boys were randomly assigned to each unit. The experimental boys were treated differently according to their interpersonal maturity levels. However, the parole revocation rates of experimental and control boys were identical at 65% during a two-year follow-up period.

The Fricot ranch study (Jesness, 1971a) was primarily motivated by staff who thought that their ability to rehabilitate delinquent boys was limited by the large 50-bed dormitories, which made establishment of close relationships between boys and staff difficult. Therefore, nearly 300 boys were randomly assigned either to a regular 50-bed unit or to an experimental 20-bed one. It is clear from the research report (Jesness, 1965) that the number of staff was the same in each unit, so that the inmate:staff ratio was much higher in the 50-bed unit.

Perhaps because of the lower inmate:staff ratio, the regime in the 20-bed unit was more informal, with five times as much contact between staff and boys, greater freedom of movement, greater emphasis on reasoning and rewards, and greater willingness of the staff to offer support and to involve themselves in the boys' problems. Nevertheless, despite promising early results, the parole revocation rate after five years was very similar for the two units, at 82% for the 20-bed unit and 90% for the 50-bed one. These high figures suggest that the disturbed young offenders in this institution were likely to reoffend no matter what treatment they were given. The parole revocation rate, therefore, is not a very appropriate measure of effectiveness. It may be that some benefits of the more relaxed, better staffed regime might have been noticeable with a more sensitive outcome measure (such as monthly arrest rates or self-reported offending).

The third important experiment carried out by Jesness (1975) was a comparison of two newly opened institutions—one operating on psychodynamic principles using group therapy and transactional analysis and the other employing a behavior modification (token economy) regime. Apart from the regimes, the institutions were very similar in organizational structure, staffing patterns, and physical layout, and over 900 boys aged 15 to 17 were randomly assigned to them. Interestingly, the parole violation rates after two years were identical in the two institutions, at 48%.

Three other institutional treatment experiments are noteworthy. The first, by Sarason and Ganzer (1973; see also Sarason, 1978) was carried out in the state of Washington, and was primarily intended to assess the efficacy of modeling as a rehabilitative tool. Nearly 200 juveniles in an institution were randomly assigned to modeling, discussion, or control groups. The aim in the modeling group was to show boys by example how to apply for a job, how to resist temptations by peers to engage in delinquent acts, how to delay gratification, and how to take problems to adults such as teachers. These kinds of problems were merely discussed in the discussion group. A five-year follow-up showed that the recidivism rates were significantly lower in the modeling and discussion conditions than in the control group.

An interesting evaluation of work release for prisoners was carried out by Waldo and Chiricos (1977) in Florida. Nearly 300 inmates were randomly assigned either to work release for two to six months or to a control group who continued to participate in other correctional programs. The two groups were comparable in many respects, including age, race, intelligence, number of prior arrests, and sentence length. This study is noteworthy for the 18 different measures of recidivism used (including self-reports of offending and arrests up to four years after release), which showed that the two groups did not differ.

One of the best known institutional programs developed in recent years is "Scared Straight" in which adult prisoners try to impress on juvenile offenders the horrors of imprisonment in an attempt to deter them from continued offending. One of these programs in California was evaluated experimentally by Lewis (1983). Over 100 male juvenile offenders were randomly assigned either to the program or to a control group. While there was no significant difference between the groups in the average number of arrests during a one-year follow-up period, more of the program juveniles were arrested (81% as opposed to 67%). These results essentially replicate those obtained in Rahway State Prison, New Jersey, by Finckenauer (1982) with a smaller sample of 81 juveniles. Similarly, in the "JOLT" (Juvenile Offenders Learn Truth) experiment in Michigan, based on 84 offenders, the small difference in reoffending rates favored the control group (Lundman, 1984). Therefore, it seems likely that contact with adult felons does not deter juveniles but makes them worse.

Taken together, these institutional treatment experiments do not give cause for a great deal of optimism about the effects of institutional programs on subsequent recidivism. The most hopeful result—by Sarason and Ganzer—suggests that a program based on modeling may be helpful, although the modeling was no more effective than discussion.

Helping Postprison Adjustment

Several experiments have been carried out to investigate the effects of special help given to prisoners to adjust in the community after leaving prison. In Copenhagen, Denmark, Berntsen and Christiansen (1965) randomly assigned over 250 prisoners either to receive special help or not. The help consisted of finding work and accommodation, financial help, assistance in straightening out difficulties with spouses and relatives, and help in negotiations with creditors and social agencies. Significantly fewer of the prisoners who received this help were reconvicted during a follow-up period of at least six years. Furthermore, the difference between the helped and control groups was greatest for those with the highest predicted probability of recidivism, suggesting that the help had been most effective with the most persistent criminals.

This experiment and the results were essentially replicated by Shaw (1974) in England. Nearly 200 male prisoners were randomly assigned either to receive special welfare help or not, and the helped group had more frequent and longer interviews with prison welfare officers. The helped group were significantly less likely to be reconvicted during a two-year follow-up period (57% as opposed to 76%), and the difference was greatest for those with the highest predicted probability of recidivism (67% reconvicted as opposed to 95% of the controls).

The reason for the success of this program is not clear. Shaw found that the helped group were not more likely to have a job or accommodation to go to than the controls, although the helped group had more favorable attitudes toward their prison welfare officers and were more likely to make contact with aftercare officers after release. The prison interviews between the helped group and their welfare officers were not particularly geared to the solution of immediate practical problems but did include long talks about them. Shaw herself thought that "the most likely way in which the experimental situation may have influenced the results was by raising the interest of the welfare officers" (p. 94). The better outcome of the helped group may possibly be a function of the better aftercare which they sought and received.

Unfortunately, Fowles (1978) attempted to replicate Shaw's results in another English prison and was unable to do so. Nearly 300 prisoners were randomly assigned to welfare officers either with a regular caseload or with a special low caseload. The helped group had an average of 10 contacts with the welfare officers during the last three months of their prison sentences, in comparison with the average 2 contacts of the controls. The helped group received more counseling and practical help and made slightly more use of aftercare officers but were not significantly less likely to be reconvicted during a one-year follow-up period.

According to Shaw (personal communication), there are two major possible reasons for the difference between the results obtained by Shaw and Fowles. One is that Shaw's prisoners were long-termers, whereas Fowles' were short-termers. It may be that help with aftercare is more important and effective for those serving long sentences. The second is that Shaw's research was carried out in the early years of the prison welfare service, when the probation officers in prisons may have been particularly keen and enthusiastic. In contrast, Fowles' experiment was conducted a few years later, after the welfare service had become more established. Clearly, a further replication is needed to decide between these two possible explanations and to establish whether this kind of help, as provided routinely in prison, is effective.

Just as varying caseloads of probation officers seemed to have little effect on recidivism, varying caseloads of parole or aftercare officers were similarly ineffective in the "Special Intensive Parole Unit" experiment of Reimer and Warren (1957). Nearly 3,800 California parolees were randomly assigned either to intensive (15-person) or regular (90-person) caseloads. There was no difference between the conditions in major arrests during a two-year follow-up period.

The tendency of ex-prisoners to relapse into crime is often attributed to their shortage of money, just as it is often supposed that much property crime is caused by economic need. Prisoners leave institutions with little money to tide them over until they can get jobs. In the United States their financial difficulties are often exacerbated by the fact that because they have been in prison, they have lost any entitlement to unemployment benefits earned in a previous employment. Rossi, Berk, and Lenihan (1980) carried out two interesting experiments designed to invetigate the effects of providing unemployment benefits for ex-prisoners after leaving institutions.

In the first ("LIFE") project, carried out in Baltimore, over 400 ex-prisoners with a high risk of recidivism were randomly assigned to receive either 13 weeks benefit or not and either job placement assistance or not. If the ex-prisoner found work, his weekly benefits were decreased from $60 to zero on a sliding scale as his weekly income increased. The results showed that the rearrest rate in one year for property crime was significantly less for those who received unemployment benefits, although this effect was not very great (22% re-arrested as opposed to 31% for those who did not receive benefits). The job placement assistance had virtually no effect.

Encouraged by the results of the LIFE experiment, the researchers embarked on the more ambitious "TARP" experiment, based on a fairly representative sample of about 4,000 prisoners released in Texas and Georgia. These ex-prisoners were randomly assigned to receive either (a) 26 weeks unemployment benefit, reduced dollar for dollar according to earnings; (b) 13 weeks benefit reduced by 100% of earnings; (c) 13 weeks benefit reduced by 25% of earnings; (d) job placement assistance only; (e) no help but the same four interviews as the previous four groups; or (f) no help and no interviews. The results of this ambitious, well-designed experiment showed that the rearrest rate in one year did not vary over the six groups in either state, suggesting that the financial aid as administered had no effect on recidivism.

The financial aid did have a significant effect in reducing the number of weeks worked, especially in the first six months of the follow-up period. As Rossi *et al.* pointed out (p. 101), "Jobs typically available to TARP members paid between $100 and $150 per week and were likely to involve unpleasant tasks. Hence, $63 or $70 per week with no work was frequently seen as better than such jobs." By means of a series of complicated analyses, Rossi *et al.* argued that the overall result showing no effect actually reflected two opposing influences that canceled each other out. Financial aid was hypothesized to have a direct effect in reducing recidivism, but it also decreased employment, which in turn led to an increase in recidivism (see also Chapter 7).

This argument seems a little contentious. The beauty of a randomized design is that it eliminates all explanations of an observed effect other than those connected with the experimentally manipulated variables. In any essentially correlational design (which is what Rossi *et al.* resorted to after the random assignment showed no effect on recidivism), it could always be argued that other unmeasured variables could explain the observed results. In the absence of an experiment demonstrating that decreased employment causes increased recidivism, the canceling out argument must remain unconvincing.

In commenting on their research, Zeisel (1982a, 1982b) argued strongly that Rossi *et al.* disregarded the crucial distinction between a controlled experiment and a correlational structural model, that the equivalence of two alleged effects was surprising, that correlational evidence (unlike a randomized experiment) required a theoretically endless chain of safeguards and assumptions to arrive at reasonably plausible causal inferences, and that nonexperimental evidence should not be used to subvert a clear experimental finding of no effect. In reply, Rossi, Berk, and Lenihan (1982, p. 393) did not entirely agree, but stated that "we would be the first to agree that . . . structural equation results are unlikely to be as convincing as results from randomized experiments." These exchanges again illustrate the importance of the experimental method in comparison with other possibilities.

The controversy surrounding the results of Rossi *et al.* has been reviewed in some detail because, as Zeisel (1982a, p. 379) pointed out, "this experiment was probably one of the best executed large-scale social experiments ever conducted in a natural setting." Despite this controversy, the results presented in this section are more encouraging than in many others. Assistance given to ex-prisoners in Denmark by Berntsen and Christiansen, in England by Shaw, and in Baltimore in the LIFE project led to decreases in recidivism. The failed replications mean that these results do not hold in all possible circumstances. Nevertheless, further experiments investigating the effects of different kinds of assistance to ex-prisoners are clearly warranted.

Police and Court Experiments

Police Experiments

In recent years, police experiments have tended to be based on areas rather than on individuals, and one of these area experiments will be discussed in the section "Experiments on Larger Units." Three experiments with individuals are worthy of note, all of them designed to study the effectiveness of different methods of police reaction to offenders.

In Blackburn, England, Rose and Hamilton (1970) compared the effectiveness of two methods of dealing with juvenile offenders, namely by a police caution only or by a caution followed by six months of police supervision. About 200 boys were randomly assigned to each condition. A two-year follow-up period showed no difference between the groups in reoffending, suggesting that the police supervision had been ineffective.

In Vancouver, Canada, Boyanowsky and Griffiths (1982) studied the effects of the appearance of police officers on the reactions of over 130 motorists stopped by them. The police officer either did or did not carry a gun and either did or did not wear reflective sunglasses, which prevented eye contact. In addition, the motorist was or was not given a ticket, but this was (presumably) not manipulated experimentally. Observers rode with the police officers and rated the reactions of the motorists who were later interviewed. Boyanowsky and Griffiths found that the motorists were more angry when the police officer was wearing a gun and also that officers wearing sunglasses were perceived as less friendly, more aggressive, and less helpful. It would be desirable to have more experiments of this kind concerned with police–citizen interaction.

In Minneapolis, Sherman and Berk (1984) compared the effectiveness of three police reaction strategies in over 300 incidents of minor domestic assault. The police officer (a) arrested the offender, or (b) ordered the offender to leave the premises for eight hours, or (c) offered advice and mediation to the participants. These strategies were randomized by the researchers. A six-month follow-up using both official records and regular telephone interviews with the victim showed that the rate of repeat incidents was lowest by a significant margin in the arrest condition. Because the offenders were rarely incarcerated after arrest for more than one week, Sherman and Berk concluded that the arrest had had an individual deterrent (as opposed to an incapacitative) effect and recommended this police reaction to domestic violence. This experiment has already provoked considerable controversy and criticism, but it is likely to be one of the most influential police research projects of the 1980s.

Although the three police reactions were randomized by the researchers, the police officers could not always carry them through successfully, for operational reasons. For example, if the offender was supposed to leave but then refused to do so or assaulted the police officer, the officer was likely to arrest the offender. This blurring of experimental conditions is not uncommon in criminological experiments, but its effects are not too serious. It means that the observed effect of any experimental manipulation is likely to be an underestimate of the true effect.

In order to preserve the benefits of randomization, it is important that comparisons be made between the originally assigned conditions rather than the finally achieved conditions. For example, in the Sherman and Berk experiment, 99% of those designated to be arrested were actually arrested, while 78% of those designated to be advised were actually advised, and 73% of those designated to be separated were actually separated. Most of those who did not receive the treatment designated in the other two conditions ended up being arrested. It is important that comparisons should be made between those designated to be arrested, advised, and separated, rather than between those actually arrested, advised, and separated. According to Sherman (personal communication), the results are essentially the same in these two comparisons.

Court Experiments

One of the most famous court experiments was the Manhattan bail project (Ares, Rankin, and Sturz, 1963). This was inspired by the belief that too few defendants were released on bail, and an attempt was made to develop a set of criteria that could guide pretrial release decisions. Defendants were interviewed about such things as their length of residence at their current address, their recent employment record, and whether they had relatives in New York City. On the basis of this information, the researchers decided whether to recommend to the court that the defendant be allowed bail.

In the case of over 700 defendants for whom release recommendations were indicated, the researchers decided at random whether to communicate this recommendation (and the information on which it was based) to the court. The recommendation had a significant effect on the court decisions; 60% of those recommended were released in comparison with 14% of the control group. Furthermore, 60% of those recommended were subsequently acquitted or had their cases dismissed, in comparison with 23% of the controls, showing the value of the pretrial release to the defendants (Botein, 1965).

Another pretrial-release experiment in New York City was carried out by Baker and Sadd (1981). Over 650 felony defendants were randomly assigned either to the Vera Court Employment Project or to a control group. Those in the project were offered vocational counseling, job training, and job placement during a four-month pretrial release period. When they appeared in court, the project workers tried to secure dismissal of their cases, and the results showed that the project was successful in getting cases dismissed. Overall, 72% of the experimental group had their cases dismissed, in comparison with 46% of the controls. However, a one-year follow-up period showed no difference between the experimental and control groups in rearrest rates or in the percentage of time employed.

A classic experiment on juvenile justice was carried out by Stapleton and Teitelbaum (1972). Following the move from a more welfare-oriented to a more legalistic juvenile court in the late 1960s, they were interested in studying the effect of providing legal representation for juvenile offenders. The experiment was carried out in two large northern urban cities, referred to as "Zenith" and "Gotham." Over 550 male juveniles in each city were randomly assigned either to be offered the services of the project lawyers (who were specially trained and had low caseloads) or to be left to the regular legal services.

The Zenith court was more legalistic in its orientation (for example, allowing tests of the admissibility of evidence and clearly separating adjudication and decision). In addition, a public defender was available in Zenith, which meant that 39% of the control group was legally represented (in comparison with 82% of the experimental group). In contrast, the Gotham court had a traditional welfare orientation. It would proceed without witnesses or a plea, it did not respect the privilege against self-incrimination, and the judge would enter a finding on different grounds from the original petition. Only 11% of the control group was legally represented in Gotham (in comparison with 83% of the experimental group).

The project lawyers were instructed to conduct themselves in an adversarial fashion and to do their best to have the case dismissed or to minimize the seriousness of the disposition. They were effective in Zenith because the experimental cases were more likely to be dismissed than the controls. However, they were ineffective in Gotham because of the welfare orientation of the judges. For example, the Gotham judges wanted the plea to serve a truth-telling function, whereas the Zenith judges treated the plea as an expression of the juvenile's desire to force the State to prove the charge rather than as a statement of fact. Consequently, more juveniles admitted the offense in Gotham than in Zenith. This experiment is interesting not only for its results, which are highly significant in relation to the key issue of due process for juveniles (see Chapter 6), but also in showing how an experimental manipulation can have different effects in different settings.

Experiments on Larger Units

Experiments can be carried out on larger units than individuals, such as areas, schools, or institutions. In practice, these kinds of units are seldom sufficiently numerous for randomization to ensure that those in each condition are equivalent. Nevertheless, experiments with larger units should be considered, and they have produced some interesting results. The best way to ensure equivalence is probably by matching, and it then becomes especially important to have measures of the dependent variable both before and after the experimental manipulation.

One of the most interesting experiments based on towns was carried out in Holland by Buikhuisen (1974). This was intended to investigate the general deterrent effect of a police and newspaper campaign on the incidence of illegally worn tires on cars. Periodically before and after the campaign, students recorded the incidence of worn tires in two towns by checking all cars parked in a representative sample of streets between 1:00 A.M. and 5:30 A.M. Fortunately for the research, few car owners in these towns had private garages. The two-week police and newspaper campaign was then mounted in one town and the other was used as a control. After the campaign, 54% of cars with worn tires had the tires renewed in the experimental town, in comparison with 27% in the control town, a significant difference. Before the campaign, the rate of renewal of worn tires was almost identical in the two towns. These results indicated that the deterrence campaign had been successful.

Interestingly, Buikhuisen then traced the owners of cars in the experimental town (using license numbers) and interviewed them. Compared with those who renewed their tires, the nonrenewers tended to be less aware of the police campaign, younger, less well educated, possessing older cars of lower value, not needing their cars for their profession, and not maintaining them adequately. Buikhuisen concluded that the campaign had been ineffective with these people because they were marginal motorists who could not really afford to have a car, let alone buy new tires.

In Finland, Tornudd (1968) also carried out an experiment based on towns and designed to investigate general deterrence. He wanted to know whether the incidence of drunkenness would decrease if offenders were less often prosecuted. Out of six towns of similar size, three were chosen arbitrarily to be experimental towns and the remaining three served as controls. In the three experimental towns, the police reduced the proportion of arrested drunks who were prosecuted and consequently fined from about 50% to about 20% over a two- to three-month period. In the control towns, the proportion fined, which was originally slightly higher than in the experimental towns at about 60%, did not change significantly. However, the experimental manipulation had no effect on the rate of arrests for drunkenness. Further research suggested that this was because the problem drinkers in the experimental towns were not aware of the change in prosecution policy.

The most famous criminological experiment based on areas is probably the Kansas City preventive patrol experiment (Kelling, Pate, Dieckman, and Brown, 1976). This was designed to investigate the effect of different levels of police patroling on crime rates. It was reported that 15 beats were randomly divided into three groups, five reactive (responding only to calls for service), five control (with one police car per beat), and five proactive (with two or three cars per beat). The three groups of beats did not differ in crimes reported either to the police or in a victimization survey, suggesting that different levels of police patroling had little effect on crime rates.

Because of the importance of this experiment, it has been subject to a great deal of critical attention. As Fienberg, Larntz, and Reiss (1976) pointed out, it seems unlikely that the beats were randomly assigned because the reactive beats were at the corners and in the middle of the experimental area. This is confirmed by Pate, Kelling, and Brown's (1975) statement that the police selected the configuration of beats that best suited the department's operational concerns. Other commentators (e.g., Larson, 1975; but see Risman, 1980) have argued that the three policing strategies were not functionally distinct.

The Newark Foot Patrol Experiment is also interesting. Police foot patrols were added in four beats that did not have them, were retained in four others, and discontinued in four others (Police Foundation, 1981). The results showed that crime rates (as measured by arrest statistics and victimization data) did not decrease in areas with foot patrols, but citizens in these areas felt more secure. Wilson and Kelling (1982) argued that the fear of crime had decreased because the patroling officers were controlling disorderly people such as panhandlers, drunks, addicts, rowdy teenagers, prostitutes, loiterers, and the mentally disturbed. Hence, the residents' beliefs that crime had decreased were not without foundation.

Clearly, more experiments on the effects of police patroling are required. It is unfortunate that the series of experiments by Schnelle and his colleagues (Schnelle et al., 1975, 1977, 1978, 1979) all involved essentially within-subjects/base-line designs rather than control groups. It is also unfortunate that most of the recent experiments based on areas cannot be found in the published literature but only in project reports. Police patroling experiments have been reviewed by Sherman (1983), and experiments on changing the physical environment by Murray (1983). It is also unfortunate that the pioneering work of researchers such as Miller (1962) and Klein (1967), who attempted to change gangs, has not been followed by controlled experiments targeted on gangs as units.

Quasi-Experiments

There are many topics that cannot be investigated experimentally, because of ethical, legal, and practical problems. In many instances, the next best way to study these topics is in a quasi-experiment. In this, a change produced by events beyond the researcher's control in nonrandomly selected groups is viewed as though some "independent" variable is influencing some "dependent" variable. Quasi-experimental analysis involves the systematic testing of alternative explanations of observed effects, or threats to internal validity, in order to establish the most likely causes (see Campbell and Stanley, 1966; Cook and Campbell, 1979).

As an example of quasi-experimental analysis, Campbell and Ross (1968) tested the hypothesis that increased penalties for speeding in Connecticut had led to a decrease in road traffic deaths. The increased penalties were indeed followed by decreased deaths, but it was then necessary systematically to test alternative explanations of this decrease. For example, could the decrease be attributed to history (events other than the crackdown), maturation (general trends over time), instrumentation (changes in recording of deaths), or instability (random variation)? Given that legal crackdowns usually followed high levels of the target social problem, could the decrease be due to statistical regression? Campbell and Ross concluded that the decrease was partly due to the crackdown, although to a considerable extent reflected instability.

Quasi-experimental analyses are especially useful in assessing the effects of new laws. For example, Ross *et al.* (1970) investigated the effect of the introduction of the breathalyzer in England on deaths and serious injuries from road accidents. After the breathalyzer was introduced, there was a 40–50% drop in casualties on weekend nights but no decrease in casualties during commuting hours. There was no change in enforcement, no general trend before the new law, no change in recording procedures, and the new law did not follow a particularly high level of road accident casualties. After reviewing a number of alternative hypotheses, Ross *et al.* were forced to conclude that the introduction of the breathalyzer had indeed caused a marked decrease in drunken driving. However, the effect was rather short lived (see also Ross, McCleary, and Epperlein, 1982).

As another example of the uses of quasi-experimental analysis, Schnelle and Lee (1974) studied the effect of a prison policy change (a decision to transfer problem inmates to an unattractive institution) on offending in a prison. The rate of offending declined after the change. The decrease could not be attributed to other events (although the change was confounded with the termination of a restricted diet), was not part of a pre-existing trend, and did not merely reflect the removal of troublesome inmates. However, it could have been due to changes in the reporting behavior of the guards or to regression (since it followed a particularly high level of offending).

As a further example, Farrington (1979b) studied the effect of official labeling (operationally defined as a first conviction) on deviant behavior (operationally defined as self-reported offending). After a conviction, self-report scores of convicted youths increased in comparison with scores of unconvicted youths. This effect could not be attributed to maturation, history, instrumentation, testing (the effect of a pretest on a posttest), regression, mortality (differential dropping out of convicted and unconvicted youths from the study), or selection (preexisting differences between convicted and unconvicted youths). Furthermore, the increase in self-reported offending seemed to follow the conviction rather than the reverse. The only remaining uncertainty was whether the conviction caused an increase in self-reporting or an increase in offending, and Farrington (1977) concluded that both were happening (see also Chapter 5).

Quasi-experimental studies can also be carried out on larger units, such as schools, correctional institutions, or even an entire correctional system. As an example, the closing of large juvenile training schools in Massachusetts in 1972 and the substitution of a network of small group homes and nonresidential programs was studied by the Center for Criminal Justice at the Harvard Law School (Miller and Ohlin, 1985). Comparison of a sample of offenders released prior to the change and those exposed to the new system showed slightly higher overall recidivism rates for those processed after the change, though lower rates were found in regions where the new system had been more fully implemented. An additional longitudinal study of a sample of youth committed under the new system revealed that the more community-based programs produced better results but that the correctional programs generally had less effect on recidivism than the postrelease experiences of the offenders with families, peers, schools, and drug use.

Conclusions in quasi-experimental analyses cannot be as convincing as those in randomized experiments. Nevertheless, quasi-experiments are far more convincing than correlational analyses and can be carried out in many instances when randomized experiments cannot. Therefore, researchers should make a greater effort to analyze nonexperimental data quasi-experimentally.

Limitations of Existing Experiments

The Dependent Variable

The major dependent variable in most existing experiments is the recidivist/ nonrecidivist dichotomy obtained from official records. This is inadequate in many respects. First of all, recidivism has a wide variety of meanings, such as police contacts, arrests, convictions, parole violation, and reimprisonment (e.g., Hawkins, Cassidy, Light, and Miller, 1977). Second, the official records reflect the behavior not only of offenders but also of official agencies. As in the argument of Lerman (1975), it is important to know if a treatment has affected crime or the reaction to crime. Third, the occurrence of one offense during a follow-up period is rather uninformative. In the past, researchers have drawn unduly pessimistic conclusions from high recidivism rates. Even if 90% of persons treated in a particular way are rearrested, this does not necessarily mean that the treatment was ineffective. The treatment might have caused a marked reduction in the frequency or seriousness of offending or in the length of the criminal career. To interpret a recidivist event as a failure implies that complete reformation is likely, whereas all the evidence from self-reported offending studies shows that offending (at least of less serious varieties) is widespread.

An implication of this last argument is that more sensitive measures of offending are needed, preferably based on interviews or observation as well as on official records. The percentage of people who become recidivists is often loosely referred to as the recidivism rate, whereas real measures of rate (offending per unit time at risk outside institutions) are required. In addition, measures of seriousness and variety of offending are needed as well as information about length of criminal career. Furthermore, because offending may be only a minor aspect of a person's life, data should be collected about other outcomes such as success in employment and personal relationships and general adjustment to the community.

Follow-up periods in experiments are often very short—between 6 months and 2 years. A longer follow-up period would make it possible to investigate the short- and long-term effects of manipulations. These are sometimes quite different. For example, in the Fricot ranch experiment (Jesness, 1971a), the juveniles housed in smaller units had a significantly lower parole revocation rate after one year but not after 5 years. Conversely, in an English comparison of eight juvenile institutions, which did not involve randomization (Dunlop, 1974), there were no significant differences in reoffending rates during the first two years of the follow-up, but differences then began to show and were quite marked by the end of 5 years. In experiments with long follow-ups (e.g., McCord, 1978; Schweinhart and Weikart, 1980), the follow-up has been after the experimental manipulation. It would be especially informative to have longitudinal data before and after, so that the impact of the manipulation could be viewed in the context of preexisting trends and the full career. Very few experiments have collected such before and after data, even in official records, although Empey and Erickson (1972) did.

Another advantage of including experimental manipulations in longitudinal studies is that the equivalence of persons in the different conditions could be investigated in detail. Also, it would be possible to study in detail the interaction between types of persons and types of treatments, which may be very important. Also, if the longitudinal study included repeated interviews, it would be possible to establish why a treatment did or did not have intended effects. The intervening variables in the chain between the independent and dependent variables are often unclear.

The Independent Variable

Most treatments in existing experiments are not based on a well-developed theory but on a vague idea about what might influence offending. The treatments given are often heterogeneous, making it difficult to know which element was responsible for any observed effect, and poorly described, making replication difficult or impossible. It is important to plan experiments so that the process, or causal chain between the independent and dependent variable, can be specified. As Sechrest and Redner (1979) pointed out, it is also important to establish if the treatment plan was carried out as intended.

Furthermore, most existing criminological experiments seem to involve manipulations that are relatively weak and unimportant. Why should anyone suppose that one or two hours a week of group counseling in a prison, for example, will make much difference to behavior outside? In a cross-sectional study of vocational training by McKee (1985), it was only prisoners who completed at least 1,000 hours of training who had significantly higher incomes on parole. In retrospect, it is not surprising that Martinson (1974) concluded that "nothing works." It is necessary to investigate the effectiveness of manipulations that can reasonably be expected to work. In addition, it is desirable to compare not just two varieties of the same treatment but two different treatments and to try to map out the dose–response relationship or the relation between different levels of a treatment and its effectiveness. Very few existing experiments have included a truly "untreated" control group, making it difficult to draw conclusions about absolute (as opposed to relative) efficacy of treatment. Rather than concluding that "nothing works," Martinson could have concluded with equal justification that "everything works equally well."

Generalization of Results

Little is known about the extent to which experimental results hold in different settings or boundary conditions or over different operational definitions of the independent and dependent variables. When an experiment is carried out in two settings, the results can be different (e.g., Stapleton and Teitelbaum, 1972), and the difference can be informative and theoretically significant.

The question of generalization is especially important in relation to small-scale pilot experiments. In theory, it would be desirable if the likely effects of large-scale social changes could be evaluated in advance in small-scale social experiments. However, the treatment staff in a small-scale experiment may be unusually enthusiastic or expert, so that the small-scale effect may not generalize to the large-scale implementation. One possible reason why LIFE was more successful than TARP (Rossi *et al.*, 1980) is because LIFE was administered by a research team and TARP by state unemployment benefit officers.

Conclusions

Randomized experiments do not show that "nothing works." They show that the effects of general help, counseling, guided group interaction, and other "talking therapies" are not notably successful with all types of offenders, but equally these methods may be successful with some types of offenders. Experiments suggest that delinquency can be prevented through preschool intellectual enrichment programs and through programs based on exposure to prosocial peers. They also suggest that juveniles can be treated effectively by behaviorally based diversion programs and by an institutional program based on modeling. Furthermore, it appears that recidivism can be reduced by giving prisoners practical help with their postprison adjustment and that domestic violence can be reduced by arresting the offenders. Admittedly, we are being optimistic in drawing these conclusions; obviously there are many negative results in the literature. However, we believe that the way forward is to build on the positive results obtained in well-designed experimental research.

Results obtained in randomized experiments in criminology have attracted a great deal of critical attention and have been very influential. The same can be said about results obtained in longitudinal studies. It is hardly an exaggeration to say that most of our firm knowledge derives from one or the other of these methods. The time is now ripe to combine them in a way that has not been attempted before. Our priorities for longitudinal–experimental research projects will be proposed in Chapter 8. Before then, we will review some of the key issues arising in the explanation, prevention, and treatment of crime to identify key questions to be investigated and to demonstrate how much our proposed projects are needed.

4
Prevention: Families and Schools

As mentioned in Chapter 2, the discovery that a small number of high-rate offenders account for a disproportionate share of arrests for serious crimes has had a major impact in recent years on the direction of criminal justice policies and research interest (Greenwood and Abrahamse, 1982). The most frequently cited statistics from the study by Wolfgang and associates of the 1945 Philadelphia birth cohort revealed that 18% of the delinquents accounted for 71% of the homicides, 73% of the rapes, 70% of the robberies, 69% of the aggravated assaults, and 52% of all arrests experienced by the cohort (Wolfgang et al., 1972). Such statistics focus attention on crime careers and the possibility of reducing crime by identifying and incarcerating the high-rate offenders; at the same time, these data raise anew the possibility of, instead, identifying these offenders at a much earlier stage and undertaking preventive measures to produce more law-abiding behavior. Accordingly, in recent years a renewed search has been activated for reliable, early signs of a potential for serious and frequent delinquent conduct. Discovery of such indicators would encourage the development of prevention programs to redirect these tendencies.

It seems natural enough that the search for early signs of troublesome behavior should focus on families and schools. These are still the basic institutions for the socialization of children, aided preferably by the back-up support of churches, neighborhood groups, and social service agencies. If it turns out that there is continuity in the development of serious delinquent and criminal careers from early evidence of socialization problems, prevention measures directed at family and school experiences may prove to be desirable and cost-effective in both human and monetary terms.

Focusing prevention efforts on the family and school is, of course, neither new nor unusual. From the attempts to create prevention programs against delinquency in the early half of the 19th century to the present, these institutions have been a central concern of reformers (Mennel, 1973). What is different now is the confidence that the increased sophistication of both theory and method in the behavioral sciences will permit a more precise determination of deficiencies in the developmental processes, which preventive programs can be designed to correct.

The Family as a Focus of Prevention Policies

The focus on the family as a target for delinquency prevention policies has been invigorated not only by the developments in research on criminal careers but also by the domination of control theory and its modifications in current explanations of delinquent conduct. In Hirschi's formulation, "Control theories assume that delinquent acts result when an individual's bond to society is weak or broken" (Hirschi, 1969, p. 16). There are four elements to this bonding: (a) attachment to the other conventional persons, (b) commitment to law-abiding conduct, (c) involvement in conventional activities, and (d) belief in the moral validity of conventional norms (Hirschi, 1969, pp. 16–39). Subsequent modifications of this theory have introduced more complex causal path models integrating other theoretical perspectives and a more prominent role for delinquent peer group influences than Hirschi thought necessary (Elliott, Ageton, and Canter, 1979; Johnson, 1979, pp. 41–70).

What is significant about control theory as an explanatory model is the major importance it attaches to the relationships of the child to parents and school authorities. The assumption is that a strong attachment to parents and teachers is necessary to curb undesirable conduct and to secure a positive set of commitments, involvements, and beliefs. A very large number of studies have been undertaken to identify those features of family life that appear most closely linked to the emergence of delinquent conduct and most likely to inhibit the formation of close family attachments. From these studies have begun to emerge a set of persistent findings of unfavorable family organization and functioning. The relevant findings from longitudinal and experimental studies have been reviewed in Chapters 2 and 3. In the following discussion we would like to highlight those results of particular importance to the development of prevention programs and further research focused on the family.

In a recent review of studies employing samples from the general population in which the family measures antedated conviction for delinquent acts, Rutter and Giller (1984, pp. 180–191) sought to identify the most important family variables associated with subsequent conviction. These include "parental criminality; poor parental supervision; cruel, passive, or neglecting attitudes; erratic or harsh discipline; marital conflict; and large family size." Though they found these variables to also be associated with nondelinquent conduct disorders, the relationships appeared to hold for delinquent conduct as well and in different cultures, ethnic groups, and social control systems. The most striking and consistent relationship of parental characteristics to delinquency was found for the variable "parental criminality." Whether this can be explained by genetics, greater police surveillance, or role modeling of aggressive and antisocial attitudes remains unresolved. Rutter and Giller also note that "parental criminality is associated with poor supervision, family discord, unemployment, reliance on welfare, and a host of other family factors which may be as important in the genesis of delinquency as the criminality per se."

Delinquency is related to intrafamily discord, as measured by a number of variables, such as quarreling, parental separations, rejection, and the escalation of hostile interactions. It is also associated with weak affectional relationships as measured by such variables as the lack of affectional identification, intimate communication, joint leisure activities, parental warmth, and acceptance of parental roles. Similarly delinquency has been associated in recent research most strongly with the extent of parental supervision coupled with the clarity of parental expectations and the efficiency of disciplinary measures. What has been most difficult, however, has been the assessment of the relative contribution of discord, weak relationships, and extent of supervision to delinquency. The overlap and interaction of the relevant dimensions of these variables confounds efforts to order priorities in devising prevention strategies.

Though Rutter and Giller (1984) note the association of socioeconomic disadvantages with the foregoing variables, they also point out that the family factors still remain crucial within different socially disadvantaged groups. They are accordingly led to stress the indirect effect of disadvantaged conditions on delinquency via the direct adverse effect on parents. They speculate that "there may be a chain of adversities which starts with socioeconomic disadvantage and which leads to the child only through the parents." The extent to which socioeconomic factors have a direct effect on the child and his delinquency remains unresolved. Similarly, the relationship between large family size and delinquency "remains somewhat of an enigma." The fact that family size and delinquency are more strongly associated in socially disadvantaged families, those with a large number of boys rather than girls, and in families showing evidence of educational backwardness suggests alternative explanations difficult to resolve.

The best evidence for this association of delinquency with various features of family life has come from longitudinal and experimental studies on which Rutter and Giller (1984) relied primarily (which we reviewed in Chapters 2 and 3). However, because the number of such studies is relatively few, a good deal of what we know is insecurely based on weaker research designs. Though more intensive research and analysis of this nature is essential in order to establish causal linkages and prevention targets with greater certainty, the persistent association of family variables and delinquency supports a major focus on the development of intervention programs to remedy critical deficiencies in family socialization processes.

Assumptions in Family Intervention Policies

A variety of different assumptions are made to support various types of family intervention programs to prevent delinquency. A comprehensive review of these assumptions would be a useful though difficult task. To test the knowledge base underlying such assumptions, it may be sufficient for our present purpose to consider three common issues and their related assumptions that typically arise in designing family prevention policies. These are (a) assumptions of continuity between early signs of trouble and later adolescent or adult crime, (b) the clarity of causal ordering in the selection of intervention strategies, and (c) the effectiveness of intervention measures.

CONTINUITY IN CONDUCT PROBLEMS

One of the basic assumptions in designing family prevention programs is that there is sufficient continuity between early troublesome conduct and later delinquency so that cost-effective measures to control delinquency can be pursued. The best support for this assumption comes from longitudinal studies that have traced such connections through adolescence to adulthood. For example, the prospective study by Farrington and West (1981) of a sample of male youth in London, England, provides striking evidence of such continuity. Poor supervision by parents, low income, parents with criminal convictions, psychomotor clumsiness, and limited vocabulary were all independently predictive of troublesomeness as rated by parents and teachers at ages 8 to 10. In turn, troublesomeness at ages 8 to 10 proved the most predictive factor for convictions at ages 10 to 13. Also in turn, conviction at ages 10 to 13 was the best predictor of self-reported delinquency at age 14 as well as conviction at ages 14 to 16. This chain of predictors from conviction at an immediately prior age to the current age category continued to hold up to the final 21- to 24-age category. Similarly, studies by Robins (1966, 1980) in the United States have found that antisocial behavior in the child is one of the best predictors of antisocial conduct in the adult, even though most of such children do not carry this problem behavior into adulthood. A number of studies have also shown that an early age of arrest for delinquency is one of the most consistent predictors of serious adolescent and adult crime (Pritchard, 1979).

The principal difficulty with the continuity assumption is that we lack sufficiently careful documentation of the linkage between troublesome behavior in the preschool years and later delinquency to support early delinquency prevention measures directed toward the family. Because only a minority of children exhibiting early conduct problems persist in exhibting the problems into later childhood and adolescence, the risk of overprediction is great and can only be avoided by the development of more reliable indicators for those problems that are likely to continue. The children who persist in frequent and serious delinquency also tend to become alienated from parents at an earlier age and to seek peer group support instead. Effective family intervention in such cases would need to occur during the childhood years and must rely on the strength of the connection between early signs of trouble and later delinquency.

CAUSAL ORDERING AND PREVENTION STRATEGIES

The selection of the most appropriate strategies for preventing delinquency by increasing family effectiveness in preventing delinquency is confounded by the difficulty in establishing causal order among the family influences leading to delinquency. It is common knowledge that growing up in families involves a constant interaction of factors with circumstances, personalities, interests, and emotions creating a complex web of actions and reactions that shape the course of conduct. Consequently, it is difficult to determine where best to intervene to redirect paths of development conducive to delinquency. For example, one of the most consistent findings of research is an association between laxness of parental supervision and delinquency (Fischer, 1983). In a study in England of an inner-city residential area and a suburban housing estate, Wilson (1980) found that parental supervision was the most important correlate of delinquency and that "the association of delinquency with laxness of parental supervision was confirmed, irrespective of place of residence and degree of social handicap" (p. 231). Whether targeting preventive programs on supervision practices would be most effective, however, is questioned by additional findings. West and Farrington's London study, for example, found that parental supervision could be dropped out of the analysis when family income and parental criminality as social handicap factors were considered and noted "the extreme difficulty of distinguishing between aspects of family life that are in practice closely interlinked" (1973, pp. 55–56). In commenting on the West and Farrington result, Wilson agreed that "the difficulty of distinguishing statistically between supervision and degree of social handicap has been an equally vexing problem in our study" (1980, p. 232). Wilson goes on to offer the following caution for those employing such findings for devising prevention strategies:

The essential point of our findings is the very close association of lax parenting methods with severe social handicap. Lax parenting methods are often the result of chronic stress, situations arising from frequent or prolonged spells of unemployment, physical or mental disabilities among members of the family, and an often permanent condition of poverty.... If these factors are ignored and parental laxness is seen instead as an "attitude" which can be shifted by education or by punitive measures, then our findings are being misinterpreted." (1980, pp. 233–234)

The issues here are important ones in considering the design of cost-effective intervention programs. For example, Wilson's findings were based on a cross-sectional analysis that made it difficult to determine whether the lax supervision by parents followed or preceded the delinquent acts. What is needed is a random allocation experimental design in the context of a longitudinal study to isolate the most strategic targets for enhancing the effectiveness of parental supervision. In Chapter 8 we offer suggestions on how this might be accomplished. Establishing a better sense of the causal order among the relevant variables should greatly improve the efficiency and cost-effectiveness of the prevention effort.

THE EFFECTIVENESS OF INTERVENTION MEASURES

The foregoing assumptions about the continuity between early troublesomeness and later delinquency and the causal ordering in the chain of influences leading to delinquency are inevitably involved in decisions relating to the design of family programs to prevent delinquency. The possibility of adding significantly to our understanding of what works to prevent delinquency would be greatly enhanced if the underlying theory and basic assumptions of intervention measures were clearly spelled out in advance of their implementation and evaluation. This would not only facilitate evaluation of the appropriateness of the measures themselves but also of the experimental and control samples and the outcome criteria for gauging impact. Often not only the theory but also the actual nature of the interventions themselves are not defined clearly enough to make definitive evaluation possible (Sechrest, White, and Brown, 1979).

In general, however, recent review of experimental projects on family prevention have yielded some cause for hope that more intensive efforts of this sort could prove effective. Farrington concluded a recent review with the following appraisal:

Delinquency prevention programmes aimed at the family seem to have a greater chance of success [than prevention projects based on counseling individual delinquents]. Binder and Newkirk (1977) describe a programme intended to change communication patterns within families, involving contingency contracting, and found lower arrest rates for the treated group. Baron, Feeney and Thornton (1973) reported a significant positive effect on delinquency of a programme based on family crisis therapy, and similar results were obtained by Alexander and Parsons (1973) with behavioural family therapy. Lee and Haynes (1980) also found a positive effect in a programme of counseling and consultation for families and schools. However, there have also been negative findings in well-designed research with family therapy. (1981, p. 7)

Further impetus to the development of family prevention programs has grown out of an increasing preoccupation in recent years with the problem of family violence (Attorney General's Task Force on Family Violence, 1984), in particular the interest in tracing the connection between various forms of child abuse (sexual, physical, emotional, and mental) and juvenile delinquency. The evidence indicates that an disproportionate number of delinquents were victims of child abuse at an early age. It has been shown through follow-up studies of abused children that a high proportion are reported as delinquent or ungovernable, surveys at youth runaway centers report a high incidence of prior abuse, and delinquents who were abused and neglected are more often involved in violent offenses (Garabino and Plantz, 1984). The link between abuse and delinquency appears strong enough to support much more careful and intensive study. Existing retrospective studies have been deficient in developing comparable data for samples of nonabused youth, and the limited number of longitudinal studies have dealt only incidentally with this linkage. There has also been a tendency to rely on self-report data, which may inflate estimates of abuse, and to use inconsistent measures of both delinquent and abusive behavior. Throughout the literature on the linkage between child abuse and delinquency, one encounters repeated recommendations to undertake a combination of longitudinal and experimental research to specify the dynamics of this relationship as well as to assess the impact of intervention (Hunner and Walker, 1981).

Perhaps the most promising set of family prevention programs to deal with the role of the family in conduct disorders has been the work of Gerald Patterson and his associates at the Oregon Social Learning Center (Patterson, 1974, 1980a).

The approach of this research group has been to focus on interactions of parents and children and to remedy deficiencies in parenting skills by prolonged training in improved child-rearing methods. Parents were taught to monitor their childrens' behavior more closely, to reach agreement on the behaviors to be rewarded or punished, to make greater use of noncoercive control measures, and to deal promptly with misconduct or emerging conflicts. The results indicated greater success in controlling aggressive behavior and some short-term beneficial effects as well with children involved in stealing. Though before-and-after measures and comparison groups were utilized in evaluating the training programs, the lack of random assignment of reasonably sized samples to control and experimental groups has limited the definitiveness of the findings. Also the training provided is intensive and costly, which may limit its more general application. Nevertheless, the results achieved thus far show sufficient promise to justify more rigorous research and development of this approach in the context of a longitudinal–experimental design along the lines we suggest in Chapter 3.

It is apparent that more careful studies are needed to evaluate and refine prevention programs directed toward the family. The results of prior studies are promising. However, we still do not know how well earlier, less serious acts of misconduct predict later delinquency; how long the beneficial effects of treatment can be sustained with sequentially less intensive treatment programs; or the feasibility of routinizing high-cost treatments that prove effective in special projects. A recent review by Loeber and Dishion (1983) concluded that deficiencies in child-rearing practices rank among the best known predictors of later delinquency. This suggests that much greater profit can be derived in this area than in others by encouraging more experimental and longitudinal research to provide better knowledge to guide the development of prevention programs.

The School as a Focus of Prevention Programs

In general, there are two major strategies employed in efforts to prevent delinquency. One focuses remedial programs on individuals identified as exhibiting early signs of disruptive behavior, maladjustment, or personal pathology. The other targets organizational reforms on agencies and institutions perceived as failing to achieve success in the socialization of children and youth.

Prevention programs centered on the educational activities of the school have traditionally favored the individual-treatment strategy. This approach has generated programs for identifying and correcting learning disabilities that may arise from physical, psychological, or social problems and that may increase the risk of delinquent conduct. The difficulty may be evident in deficiencies of hearing, vision, nutrition, or learning skills. There may be evidence of child abuse or neglect, lax parental control and supervision, or family disorganization. The child's behavior may exhibit ungovernability through disobedience and lack of respect for adult authority, drug abuse, truancy, disorderly classroom conduct, fighting, or destruction of property.

In response, schools have employed social case work methods, counseling for children and parents, remedial training in educational skills, and various disciplinary measures including the threat of suspension, expulsion, or referral to juvenile court. Considering the number and variety of individually oriented prevention efforts initiated by the schools, there are surprisingly few major evaluation studies of their effectiveness. In general, the findings have been discouraging though not conclusive. In Chapter 3, we reviewed the results of two school experiments in delinquency prevention. The study by Meyer *et al.* (1965) involved the random assignment of 400 girls in a vocational high school to an experimental group receiving social case work assistance or to a control group. The researchers concluded that this type of intervention had no significant effect on delinquency. Similarly, a study by Reckless and Dinitz (1972) of the random assignment of 1,000 boys, regarded as most vulnerable to delinquency, to regular seventh-grade classes or to experimental ones involving remedial reading and the presentation of appropriate role-model material proved ineffective in preventing delinquency or improving the self-concept of the boys.

In recent years, however, the focus of school experiments in delinquency prevention has shifted toward an exploration of organizational change strategies. This interest has been stimulated by the efforts of educators to identify the organizational characteristics of effective as compared to ineffective schools. The underlying assumption has been that schools that are effective in holding student interest and producing high levels of scholastic achievement will also be effective in preventing delinquency. Unfortunately, only a few studies have included subsequent delinquency as a measure of effectiveness along with educational achievements.

Perhaps the most influential study, which did include the delinquency variable, is that undertaken by Michael Rutter and his associates (Rutter, Maughan, Mortimore, and Ouston, 1979) of 12 inner-city secondary schools in London. The relative effectiveness of the schools was measured by attendance, pupil misbehavior in school, delinquency, and achievement scores on public examinations. As one might expect, delinquency correlated highly with attendance (.77), academic outcome (.68), and school misbehavior (.72) (p. 93). The authors were able to rule out individual intake measures such as pupil behavior and achievements in primary school and social background factors as explanations of the marked variation among the schools on the various types of outcome. Instead they concluded that "in a part of inner London known to be disadvantaged in numerous ways, some schools were better able than others to foster good behavior and attainments" (Rutter *et al.*, 1979).

Rutter and his associates carried the analysis further by trying to identify those characteristics of the schools that might account for the variations in outcome measures. They were unable to find significant associations with physical or administrative features of the schools such as size of school or classes, age of building, overcrowding, schools with religious affiliation versus local authority maintenance, and sex composition (though, of course, the girls' schools had lower delinquency rates). The authors cautioned that the small number of schools (nine including boys) made the comparative conclusions quite tentative.

The second set of organizational characteristics measured the association with outcome of various features of the school and its operation, under the designation "school processes." These concerned variations among the schools in such aspects as relative emphasis on academic matters, actions taken by teachers in conducting lessons, rewards and punishments, learning conditions established for the pupils, children's responsibilities and participation in school activities, the stability of teaching and friendship groups, and staff organization. These features of school processes were examined individually and then combined to examine the correlations with outcomes. The results showed a consistent and very strong correlation between the overall school process scores and pupil conduct within the school (.92) and a relatively high correlation with academic achievement (.76), while the relation to attendance (.65) and delinquency (.68) were lower though still significant (Rutter et al., 1979, pp. 142–143). Though these findings are limited by the small number of schools (eight) on which the correlations are based, they do indicate that it is possible to identify specific features of school organization that are strongly and consistently associated with important outcomes such as academic performance, attendance, behavior, and delinquency. They offer useful suggestions of the types of experiments that can be conducted to test under more controlled conditions the causal effect of school processes on desired outcomes.

The study by Rutter and his associates also attempted to examine the effect of external ecological factors on differences in the schools. However, as a result of the particular inner-city districts chosen for study, "most of the children came from socially disadvantaged clusters" (1979, p. 148). Though the 11 clusters of ecological areas showed small variations in delinquency rates, those rates were not statistically significant. The authors concluded that the areas may have influenced outcomes in some small way but could not account for the school variations in outcomes.

The study did succeed, however, in showing a close relationship between delinquency and attendance and what they categorized as "academic balance." Delinquency rates were lower and attendance higher when schools had a relatively high concentration of students in the upper ability groups at intake. Rutter et al. attributed this to a collective or group effect capable of creating a better context for learning. Though the individual elementary achievement scores at intake to secondary school did not account completely for differences among the schools in outcomes, schools with a low proportion of more able students at intake tended to exhibit high delinquency, low attendance, and, to a lesser extent, poor academic attainment. In contrast, the correlations of the academic balance variable with pupil behavior in school and with the composite social process score were not significant. The authors suggest the possibility that peer group influences on delinquency and attendance may be sensitive to the climate created by concentrations of low- or high-ability groups, whereas pupil behavior in school is more responsive to features of school organization as reflected in the social process variable (Rutter *et al.*, 1979, pp. 153–160).

The results of this comparative study of inner-city London secondary schools have important policy implications for delinquency prevention. They suggest a series of actions within the jurisdictional capacity of school authorities to shape the social processes of school life and the mix of ability groupings so as to produce more favorable outcomes in achievement, attendance, in-school behavior, and delinquent tendencies. The authors note that their study benefited from the availability of longitudinal data, which enabled them to control for pupil characteristics at intake and to relate outcomes to experiences within the secondary school context. They also note the need for experimental studies to fix the direction of causal influences as a guide to policy decisions.

We have suggested that there is a causal relationship between school process and children's progress. Firm conclusions about causation can only come from controlled experimental studies. The only way to be sure that school practices actually influence children's behaviour and attainments is to alter those practices and then determine if this results in changes in the children's progress. (Rutter *et al.*, 1979, p. 180)

This interest in identifying the organizational characteristics of schools that are effective in advancing educational achievement and in reducing pupil misbehavior, absenteeism, and delinquent conduct has also been fostered by an increasing concern with violence and theft within the school environs. A recent review by Jackson Toby (1983a) of national survey data in the United States on school crime and violence indicated how serious and pervasive the problem has become. Survey data gathered in 1976 showed that larceny and theft of property far exceeded the rates of assault and robbery, and the highest rates occurred in junior rather than senior high schools, especially in large cities. Nevertheless, Toby concluded that "at least half the junior high school students in schools in the largest cities were assaulted and a third were robbed each year. . . . (whereas) perhaps 10 percent of junior high school teachers in the largest cities were assaulted and 5 percent were robbed during the school year" (1983a, p. 9). Though it appears in large cities that trespassers or intruders from the community account for most of the crimes of rape, robbery, and larceny with contact, enrolled students figured more prominently in assaults and larceny without contact. In all likelihood, the anonymity of large city schools results in a number of crimes by enrolled students being attributed instead to unknown intruders. Nevertheless, the sheer volume of crime induces a fear of violence among both teachers and students that seriously inhibits successful education. Because some schools are more effective than others in controlling school crime, the problem again becomes one of trying to identify the relevant characteristics of these effective schools and experimenting with organizational reforms to implement them more widely. In the following section, we will explore briefly some of the recent proposals for such changes and the major assumptions and evidence on which they rest.

Issues in School Organizational Reforms

There have been many proposals for changing school procedures and organization to increase the educational achievements of students that might also serve to reduce or redirect delinquent tendencies. For our present purpose we shall consider several major proposals in which preventing delinquency is an explicit objective.

SEGREGATING THE TROUBLEMAKERS

In his review of school violence, Jackson Toby noted that there are natural processes at work distributing students and teachers between effective and ineffective secondary schools in large city systems: "As a result of natural processes of social competition in big-city school systems, the least troublesome students with the best academic skills, the more stimulating teachers, and the more competent principals gravitate to one group of high schools, and badly behaved students, demoralized teachers, and administrative hacks gravitate to another" (1983a, p. 36). Once this process gets underway it is difficult to stop. Two alternative strategies have been attempted, neither of which appears wholly satisfactory. One is to redistribute the troublesome students throughout the system by setting quotas for each school. As Toby observes, this policy will elicit strong opposition from parents seeking to protect a superior school, refusing to permit their children to be transferred to an inferior one. Strong political pressures develop in these large city systems for protecting the integrity of the selective, elite schools where high educational performance is expected. Furthermore, spreading the troublemakers around may simply diffuse the violence, lower educational standards, and encourage movement to suburban or private schools.

The other option is to pursue the obverse policy—facilitating this selectivity by concentrating the troublemakers in special schools. Toby suggests that this has proved more feasible historically. The excellent schools are protected, and, even in the substandard schools, classification of students into different vocational and academic tracks creates "islands of academic achievement and safety" (1983a, p. 42). This policy also has its political hazards because it can result in trapping many students from economically disadvantaged families and racially segregated neighborhoods of the city in these schools. The concentration of educationally unmotivated or emotionally disturbed youth in special schools might make their successful learning or escape progressively more difficult as time goes by. Assignment to such schools is likely to have a deleterious labeling effect and to create a self-fulfilling expectation of failure that would increase crime rather than prevent it (see Chapter 8).

Toby's preferred solution is to establish minimum behavioral standards for being allowed to remain enrolled in school. Such a policy would require change in the attendance laws, perhaps lowering the compulsory age to 14 or 15 (1983a, pp. 42–45). Youth who are not motivated to fulfill minimum educational standards for attendance, who engage in disruptive conduct, and who do not attend to educational tasks would be dismissed but permitted to return when ready to meet these standards. As the trend toward continuing education for adults expands, increasing opportunities would be available for the resumption of education at older ages. Removal of the unmotivated would be expected to create a more favorable educational climate for those who remain. There are, of course, potential pitfalls here as well. Such a policy may lead school authorities to relax efforts to awaken a commitment to education in youth from disadvantaged backgrounds, where the fruits of education are less obvious or less valued. The release of youth from compulsory schooling does not make them prepared to compete for legitimate employment, however. Toby suggests alteration of the minimum wage laws for youth to open up more employment opportunities (1983b, pp. 84–86). It is also possible, of course, that more of these youth who are not attending school will turn to crime as a career.

What is apparent from this discussion of ways to improve the educational climate of schools, to reduce school violence, to deal more successfully with educationally disruptive youth, and to prevent delinquency through school reorganization is the need for more experimentation with alternative policies and careful evaluation of their effectiveness so that the longer-term consequences are also factored in. Thinking about the strengths and weaknesses of policy alternatives involves many assumptions of fact and theory for which carefully designed experiments in the context of longitudinal studies can provide evidence and a more solid basis for choosing among them.

PRESCHOOL PROGRAMS

Among the social reforms initiated in the decade of the 1960s, one of the most prominent was the Head Start Program. It was based on the observation that children who had been exposed to preschool programs showed improved cognitive development, attentiveness, and learning skills on school entry that led to higher levels of educational achievement. The Head Start Program sought to extend these benefits to disadvantaged children who ordinarily would not have had access to this preparatory opportunity. As we noted in Chapter 3, the Consortium for Longitudinal Studies reported follow-up results of these programs in a 1983 report. The results showed beneficial effects over the long term especially in the increased rate of high school graduation and a decreased rate of special education placements. Unfortunately, data on delinquency was not routinely collected along with the measures of school success.

The one carefully designed Head Start project to collect delinquency data was carried out in Michigan and reported by Schweinhart and Weikart (1980). As we noted in Chapter 3, the program was targeted on disadvantaged black children and involved assignment to experimental and control groups. In addition to superior academic performance by the experimental group, who received a preschool intellectual enrichment program, the results showed less misbehavior in school and lower rates of self-reported delinquency and serious delinquent behavior. These findings suggest that preparatory experiences can not only make the early school years more rewarding but also that the benefits continue to be evident throughout and even after the school years, affecting the likelihood of involvement in delinquent conduct either inside or outside the school environment. The consistency of the results on school success in the Michigan study and other experimental Head Start programs suggests the desirability of gathering delinquency data for these other programs as well in order to confirm or qualify the findings of the Schweinhart and Weikart study. In addition, the positive results thus far suggest the desirability of further experimentation and follow-up of the effect of preschool programs with more careful attention to the potential delinquency prevention payoffs.

OTHER PROPOSED SCHOOL REFORMS

The comparative studies of school effectiveness are generating ideas for making the organization of schools more conducive to successful learning and more capable of preventing delinquency. Unfortunately, the failure to collect data on delinquency as well as school achievement has seriously limited evaluation of the preventive effect of these proposed reforms. For example, a study by Edmonds and Frederiksen (1978) on effective schools for poor children in urban areas emphasized the importance of strong administrative leadership, a climate of expectation of successul achievement, a clear predominance of educational over other school activities, and frequent monitoring of the progress of the students. It would appear that reforms conducive to meeting such standards would also aid in preventing delinquency, but we are not yet certain of the relative importance of the proposed reforms for prevention. Similarly, Slavin's (1980) studies at the Center for Social Organization of Schools (Johns Hopkins University) have demonstrated the value of introducing cooperative learning techniques in classrooms formerly organized on individual competition principles. The organization of mixed ability teams enlists peer group support for educational attainment, while still permitting both group and individual grading of performance. Again what is needed is the inclusion of delinquency prevention objectives and measures.

The research program of the Center for Social Organization of Schools does include studies of the effects of school on delinquency and evaluation of delinquency prevention programs. Though this work is still in progress, it provides an example of the kind of focus needed to assess the effect of school reforms on delinquency. The approach taken is similar to that advocated in a technical assistance monograph released by the Office of Juvenile Justice and Delinquency Prevention of the U.S. Department of Justice (1982).

Organizational change is considered to be the most promising and cost-effective strategy possible on the basis of current state-of-the-art findings. . . . These strategies require initiatives grounded in schools, work, families, and neighborhoods. Such strategies involve a reordering of the ways in which institutions [e.g., schools] operate in providing services that fall within their mandate and community responsibility. The emphasis is on changing the attitudes, management, and practice of service delivery within community organisations. (p. 48)

This policy was heavily influenced by a report from the Center for Action Research based in Boulder, Colorado. This report made the following observation and recommendation:

For a significant body of students, the values emphasized, the social structure, and the social interactions of schools compose a pattern of reinforcements by which these students learn that what they are about is not valued, that they [and those they come to associate with] are not expected to do much of worth and are not going to go very far and, when they get there, it will not amount to much. They learn that there is not much for them in schools. Their stake in, and possibilities for, conventional and productive action are eroded; their risk of delinquency is increased. They learn that, if they are to get what is valued, they may have to violate the rules, and they learn that there are others like them who will support them in that approach.

The intent of the recommendations made is to change that pattern of reinforcements. Values are to be realigned and differently emphasized so that more youth can make a connection of importance and relevance to the schools. The structures of the school are to be rearranged so that more students can demonstrate competence and learn that they are competent and can belong. Greater participation of the school in the community and of the community in the school makes available a greater array of attractive models to emulate. Rearrangement of evaluation procedures such as grading increases the probability of social rewards for performance and increases the probability that a commitment and attachment to schooling and to conventional kinds of behaviour will be learned. The outcomes of such changes in schools should include more effective socialization to conventional behaviour, improved self-concept and internal controls, reduced alienation, and a reduction in delinquent behaviour. (Johnson, Bird, Little, and Beville, 1981)

In a recent review of this policy position, David Farrington (1985) took issue with the rather complete and somewhat cavalier rejection of individual treatment and remedial programs targeted on troublesome or delinquent youth. This rejection of individually oriented programs is neither justified nor necessary at this stage of development. There is a need to explore both individual and organizational approaches. Recently a start has been made on organizational research of sufficient promise to justify its expansion through more carefully designed longitudinal–experimental studies. The pursuit of this objective should not preclude continuation of individually oriented treatment experiments as well.

A large-scale experiment to test the effect of school-based reforms on delinquency prevention was undertaken in 1981 as a collaborative project between the National Center for the Assessment of Delinquent Behavior and Its Prevention, at the University of Washington in Seattle, and the Westinghouse National Issues Center in Columbia, Maryland (Weis, Janvier, and Hawkins, 1981). The prevention project was directed toward randomly selected junior high school students in six east coast cities over a two-year period. It was designed to implement six program elements requiring various degrees of change. "These six program elements include management of change, schools-within-a-school, orientation of the curriculum, methods of instruction, student involvement, and school/family programs" (Weis *et al.*, 1981, p. 3). In addition, a more intensive and comprehensive approach was planned for Seattle, Washington. The Seattle project includes all the elements to be implemented in the other six sites as well as additional interventions directed toward families, peers, and the community. It was planned to target elementary school students as well as middle and senior high school students and to assess the results over a 10-year period instead of over 2 years.

This is a very complex project involving many program elements especially in the comprehensive design for Seattle. It does offer much promise, however, through the proposal of a longitudinal–experimental design and its capability of assessing the separate and cumulative preventive effect of the program elements. The future of this ambitious project, however, is still in doubt due to an interruption in funds occasioned by a shift in policy objective of the funding agency. The design of the project and its evaluation procedures, nevertheless, may provide a useful model for experimentation and evaluation of the effect of organizational change in the basic socializing agencies for youth.

It is apparent in the foregoing discussion of family and school delinquency prevention programs that these institutions are of critical importance as targets of prevention efforts. The undeniable importance of the family and school in the socialization of youth accords them a central role in any comprehensive prevention program. Many useful studies and proposals have been made, but we are at the stage where progress in the development of effective prevention policies requires more carefully designed experimentation and evaluation to sort out the most strategic targets and procedures to be pursued.

5
The Effects of Labeling

Deeply embedded in the criminal law is the assumption that the punishment specified for criminal acts reflects communal condemnation of these acts as well as an effort to control their future occurrence. Adjudication of guilt and imposition of sanctions consequently attach a criminal label and a social stigma that reflects this condemnation. One of the most influential criminological theories of the last 20 years has been labeling theory, which focuses on this process and raises important questions about it. How do particular acts become defined as criminal or deviant? What takes place in the process by which labels and stigma are successfully imposed? What effect does labeling have on the subsequent conduct of offenders or deviants? In this chapter we will focus on the policy issues raised by this last question.

From the earliest times, authorities have counted on the stigmatizing effect of punishments as retribution and deterrence for criminal or deviant acts. Visible disfigurements such as branding with a hot iron or cutting off fingers, hands, nose, or ears were intended as permanent public signs of an inferior status arising from wrongdoing. Today a less drastic functional equivalent is sought through public notice and establishment of a public record of arrests, charges, trials, convictions, and sentences for criminal offenses. Only in juvenile court proceedings has an effort been made to mitigate this labeling effect by restricting public notice of arrests and maintaining the confidentiality of the adjudication and disposition decisions and the resulting delinquency record. These efforts at mitigation were a direct outgrowth of the philosophical premises of the juvenile court movement which sought treatment rather than punishment in the best interests and needs of the child in a civil instead of criminal proceeding. Current efforts to reexamine and redefine the mission of the juvenile court are discussed more fully in Chapter 6, but it is already apparent that the confidentiality of the juvenile record and court processes are being challenged as appropriate policies. It is therefore timely to consider the current state of the evidence on the assumptions contained in labeling theory as it applies to the control of juvenile and adult crime.

At the level of policy formulation, labeling theory gives rise to two contending positions on the effects of labeling. On the one hand, proponents point to the important contribution that the stigmatizing effect of criminal justice processing makes in deterring potential offenders who may still have some stake in a law-abiding style of life. On the other hand, opponents of labeling practices point to the restrictions on law-abiding opportunities for stigmatized offenders, which might drive them deeper into involvement with criminal associates and add their number to the ranks of those high-rate offenders committed to a life of crime. Proponents of labeling are focusing on the general and specific deterrent effects; opponents are focusing on the pressure toward careers in crime. At the present time the available evidence suggests that each of these positions has merit. The problem of policy formulation on this issue may be less a choice of one position over another than it is a question of how to maximize some effects and minimize others. For example, before current efforts to restructure or eliminate the juvenile court reach fruition, it is important to consider what more we need to know to deal with this policy problem.

The Process of Labeling

In common parlance, the terms *criminal* and *delinquent* are often loosely used to condemn acts of which we strongly disapprove. However, the successful labeling of offenders as criminal or delinquent requires the initiation of a process leading to a finding of culpability in a juvenile or adult court. In a seminal article, Harold Garfinkel (1956) has described this process from a social point of view as a ceremony of status degradation. The process of determining guilt and sentence implicitly or explicitly entails a ritual of denunciation that recharacterizes the offender as a person of lower status, deserving of public condemnation. In theory this process is most successful when the offender's total identity is reconstituted so that "what he is now is what, 'after all', he was all along" (Garfinkel, 1956). The offender is now a murderer, rapist, robber, or thief and not a law-abiding citizen deserving of trust and respect.

Labeling theory has gained prominence in recent years because it describes an interactive process that is more or less subject to official or public control. It focuses attention not only on what the offender has done but on the moral indignation this act arouses in others and the actions taken to attach stigma and to modify or confirm it subsequently. The theory is a natural development in a more general body of social theory known as "symbolic interactionism." The founders of this perspective in social psychology were trying to understand the process by which a self-conception emerges in the socialization of the child (Cooley, 1902; Mead, 1918, 1934). They theorized that the conception of self arises and is objectified through a process of interaction between the child and significant other persons in his life in which the child learns to take the position of the other toward his own acts. In play, the child adopts different roles and eventually internalizes this role-taking to control his conduct in relation to the anticipated reactions and expectations of others. Since this process is a continuing one, the theory of labeling seeks to understand what effect the attachment of criminal definitions has on self-conception and future conduct.

In large part, the theory of labeling has been developed through study of the process by which noncriminal forms of behavior become defined as deviant and lead to the acceptance of a deviant identity. Thus, for example, studies have been conducted from this perspective on homosexuality, alcoholism, prostitution, and mental illness. But the theory has also been extended to studies of the process of acquiring a delinquent or criminal identity and self-conception. In this connection, it would appear that the definition of conduct as delinquent or criminal is less problematic than in the case of consensual or victimless offenses. However, the process of decriminalizing some forms of conduct and criminalizing others is a recurring one reflective of changes in the social, economic, and moral development of society. For example, prostitution, homosexuality, abortion, and status offenses for youth have been decriminalized in some states, while newly emerging threats to public safety, such as environmental pollution, have acquired criminal sanctions. In addition, the Marxist-oriented radical criminology literature of recent vintage has sought to describe the definition of crimes as a direct reflection of the prevailing power structure of the society (Greenberg, 1981).

The labeling theory literature has been more useful to criminologists in understanding the selective processes of law enforcement and criminal justice and their effect on the offender. Studies of the police handling of delinquent or disruptive youth, for example, indicate that the decision to warn, refer, or arrest may sometimes depend as much on a youth's attitude, demeanor, and deference to authority as it does on the nature of the offense and the strength of the evidence, especially for minor crimes (Piliavin and Briar, 1964). Labeling theory is concerned with identifying the criteria invoked to classify offenders for official action, the measures employed to attach labels, and the effect of the labeling process on an offender's self-conception and future conduct (Lemert, 1951, 1967). Of most interest in the present context are the responses of offenders and others to the labeling process.

Responses to the Labeling Process

Some criminologists concerned with the development of delinquent and criminal careers have stressed the importance of labeling and stigmatization in this development. Frank Tannenbaum characterized this process as one involving the "dramatization of evil."

The person becomes the thing he is described as being. Nor does it seem to matter whether the valuation is made by those who would punish or by those who would reform. . . . The harder they work to reform the evil, the greater the evil grows under their hands. The persistent suggestion, with whatever good intentions, works mischief, because it leads to bringing out the bad behavior that it would suppress. The way out is through a refusal to dramatize the evil. (1938, pp. 19–20)

In a further elaboration of this process Edwin Lemert noted:

The deviant person is one whose role, status, function and self-definition are importantly shaped by how much deviation he engages in, by the degree of its social visibility, by the particular exposure he has to the societal reaction, and by the nature and strength of the societal reaction. (1951, pp. 22–23)

The initial acts of deviance that result in successful labeling of the offender have been conceptualized as "primary deviation." Once the label is attached, a new situation is created for the offender in which he must deal with all of the constraints and reactions attached to a person occupying this deviant role. The deviant acts and social definitions that result from his efforts to cope with the constraints, stigma, and problems of this role have been defined as "secondary deviation" (Lemert, 1967). One possible development in this situation is that the deviant's self-conception becomes wholly dominated by the requirements of this role. Schur (1971) has described this condition as "role engulfment" and defines it as

the tendency of the deviator to become "caught up in" a deviant role, to find that it has become highly salient in his overall personal identity (or concept of self), that his behavior is increasingly organized "around" the role, and that cultural expectations attached to the role have come to have precedence, or increased salience relative to other expectations, in the organization of his activities and general way of life. (p. 69)

It is important to remember, however, that the process of labeling is an interactive one and that the defined deviants are not simply passive objects molded and shaped by societal reactions to their conduct. Some may accept the deviant identity and become immersed in a deviant subculture that tolerates and even supports their deviance. Others will seek ways to disavow their deviance. Such different responses raise a number of empirical questions. How are responses affected by the circumstances of the labeling process such as the nature of the offending act, the types of persons involved in attaching the label, and the amount of public visibility and knowledge of the sanctions imposed? What types of defenses are employed by those labeled? How are responses affected by differences in personality, background, and prior experience? To what extent can increases or decreases in deviant conduct be traced to the effect of the labeling process?

It is the issue of the effect of labeling in increasing deviant conduct that has caused the most controversy among criminologists. Labeling theory has been attacked on the grounds that it does not lead to theoretical propositions that can be readily tested by empirical research studies. Attempts to formulate such propositions and to examine the relevant empirical evidence from research studies have sometimes lent support to labeling theory (Black and Reiss, 1970; Lemert, 1976; Lundman, Sykes, and Clark, 1978) but more often have been assessed as discrediting the effect of labeling as a factor in increasing delinquent or criminal conduct (Wellford, 1975; Tittle, 1980b; Hirschi, 1980). That this issue has not been fully resolved is evident from continuing efforts to explore the responses of offenders to stigmatizing definitions of their conduct in recent research studies.

Some Research Findings

In an effort to determine the effects of labeling, Farrington reexamined the Cambridge study data from this theoretical perspective (see also Chapter 3) (Farrington, 1977, 1978b). He established that a first conviction led to higher self-reported delinquency scores in subsequent years whether reconvictions occurred or not, though those convicted had higher scores generally. The first conviction seems to be a crucial turning point because those receiving only police cautions were not significantly different from those with no police cautions or convictions. Farrington concluded that these results lend support to the theory that labeling, as evidenced by an official conviction for an offense, has a "deviance amplification" effect as compared to those reporting delinquent acts who were not convicted. The analysis also showed that youth convicted prior to age 14 had higher delinquency scores at ages 14 and 18 than those first convicted in later years, but they reported a greater decrease in delinquency by age 21, whether institutionalized at some stage or not. Unfortunately the available data were insufficient to make clear why this should be so. The Cambridge study data also permitted an exploration of changes in attitude toward the police following a first conviction. The findings revealed the development of more hostile attitudes toward the police after a first conviction and a significant correlation of these attitudinal changes and delinquency scores. Apparently "increases in delinquent behavior were accompanied by increases in aggressive attitudes," but the aggressive attitudes show no change in later years when delinquencies decreased (Farrington, 1978b).

In several studies Gold and his associates (Gold and Williams, 1969; Gold, 1970; Miller and Gold, 1984) demonstrated that the penetration of youth into the juvenile justice system appeared to result in increased delinquency compared to youth involved in comparable offenses who were not apprehended. In the most recent study (Miller and Gold, 1984), those processed by the official systems tended to exhibit more serious subsequent offenses but no significant difference in frequency from those not apprehended. The experience of official processing appeared to have psychological effects displayed by a worsening of attitudes toward school and in a diminished sense of personal well-being, but there were no significant differences between those apprehended and those not apprehended in their perception of being labeled by parents and teachers. Thus direct evidence that official processing produced more serious delinquencies compared to those not apprehended could not be acquired by the measures employed in the study.

That the labeling effect of official action is still disputed in current research is also evident in two studies comparing this effect on status offenders and delinquents. The first study by Thomas in Virginia, of appearances and reappearances of juveniles before a juvenile court, found that status offenders were more likely than delinquents to reappear in juvenile court—a finding interpreted as contrary to labeling theory assumptions (Thomas, 1976). A more recent study in Michigan reached the opposite conclusion in finding that status offenders reappeared in court with the same frequency as those initially charged with felonies or misdemeanors but for less serious offenses on second and subsequent appearances (Kelly, 1983). Furthermore, seriousness of offense increased for both status and delinquent offenders on subsequent reappearances, a finding interpreted as representing an effect partly attributable to the stigmatizing consequences of official processing and punishment. In both of these studies again the labeling effect is inferred from official actions rather than directly observed or measured. There is a need for more careful study of the process of labeling and the responses to it in order to clarify the different effects noted in such studies.

These studies suggest, however, a complex process in operation with many trade-offs depending on individual circumstances and resources for coping with the labeling effect. One approach has been to examine the degree of intimacy or social distance between the convicted offender and those reacting to him. Detailed interviews and observations of a sample of 45 persons with no prior institutional experience who spent four months in confinement showed that "the more socially distant a person is, the greater the likelihood that he will treat the ex-inmate as fundamentally stigmatised" (Ericson, 1977). The more information others have about the offender through prior intimate contact, the less likely they are to stereotype the offender in terms of his criminal conviction and confinement. For example, family members are likely to have a stake in normalizing the situation and helping the offender to gain a more conventional identity in order to reduce the stigma attached to the family as a result of his conduct. They are also aware of many other social facts about the offender that permit them to perceive the criminality as uncharacteristic of his "true" identity. Ericson's study also found that the greatest tolerance and acceptance of the offender as essentially unstigmatized occurred among close friends. In contrast, the greatest stigmatizing effect was displayed by new employers and the police and, to a surprising extent, by probation officers because of the tendency of the control function to dominate the obligation to assist reintegration.

A more recent study confirms these results but carries the analysis further by examining the significance and credibility of the labeler from the perspective of the offender (Morash, 1982). The subjects were 201 randomly selected white males between 14 and 16 years of age charged with adult-type misdemeanors in Anne Arundel County, Maryland. As one might expect, "parents and friends were relatively high in both credibility and significance to the youths... [while] ...adult neighbors, and particularly police, were low...." (Morash, 1982, p. 80). Since both parents and friends are seen as more significant (in the sense that the youth cares more about what they think of him) and more credible (because they have a truer picture of what he is really like), their reactions are likely to have a more profound effect on the youth's positive or negative self-conception. The tendency of youths to defend a positive self-concept is apparent in their tendency to discount more negative labelers as less credible and significant. The least easily dismissed were the negative labels conferred by friends. The most delinquent youths were more likely to discount and to care less about how police and adults saw them. In addition, this study explored the effect of formal versus informal procedures by randomly assigning youths either to a public, court-like procedure, run by the Community Arbitration Program, or to the traditional, informal court intake hearing. The idea was to test whether more formal procedures had a more negative labeling effect. The findings disclosed that "the more formal procedure resulted in somewhat more perceived negative labeling by the person presiding over the hearing. . . . However, the presiding person was considered to be somewhat less credible" (Morash, 1982, p. 83).

Though more rigorous experimental and longitudinal research designs are needed, as this study notes, to explore the longer-term effects of these processes on delinquent conduct and to take account of other labeling effects, such as the effect on future decisions of the criminal justice system, the study concludes with some suggested implications:

The practical implication of the study is that diversion from juvenile justice procedures without simultaneous attention to juveniles' relationships with other people will probably not have particularly desirable effects on the juveniles' self-concepts. The serious delinquents will continue to see other adults, such as parents, as insignificant. Thus, they will have no incentive to avoid negative labeling in the future.

A failure to divert will probably not harm the self-concept of most infrequent delinquents, since they tend to regard contradictory positive labeling by other adults, such as parents, as coming from significant sources. Therefore, it seems that most infrequent delinquents would tend to neutralize negative labels and/or change their future behavior to conform with their own relatively positive self-concepts and the expectations of others. Moreover, youths seem to have their own capacities to remain insulated from negative labels.

In light of study findings, a major issue in design of juvenile justice procedures and related diversion programs is the potential for improving delinquents' regard for other people who matter and who are a legitimate influence. The possible negative effects on self-concept of labeling by justice employees appear to be a less critical problem. (Morash, 1982, p. 86)

From the foregoing reports it is apparent that more intensive analysis is needed within the same study, not only of the labeling process itself—including the defenses that offenders are able to raise to neutralize the stigmatizing effect—but to the effects of official sanctions on future conduct. The value of coupling such a study of process with the outcome of sanctions is demonstrated by the insights gained in a recent longitudinal study of drug dealing. The study gathered data over a six-year period through extensive contacts and interviews with 34 respondents involved in middle-level drug dealing (Ekland-Olson, Lieb, and Zurcher, 1984). It focused on the way in which the organization of interpersonal ties and networks affected the perception and fear of official sanctions, and it found that the fear of sanctions in the initial stages of drug dealing depended on the effect sanctions would have on the value attached to relationships with conventional persons. With greater involvement in drug dealing, such ties tended to weaken and ties to other dealers to strengthen so that the fear of a stigmatizing effect was reduced. As interpersonal ties became more constrained and limited by the fear of disruption through arrest and punishment, the reliance on a denser and more enclosed network of relationships intensified. Suspicion of strangers as possible undercover agents, or potential informants, limited activity to those buyers deemed safe within the network. The stigmatizing effect of official sanctions was mitigated by tolerance and support within those networks of the drug-dealing activity. But the fear of stigma was replaced by the fear that sanctions would disrupt the network of relationships on which successful dealing depended. This fear of sanctions thus restricted the maintenance of "weak" ties and of "bridging" ties to potential markets. Paradoxically, the study notes that it also limited access to legitimate opportunities that might substitute for drug dealing. It served to strengthen adherence to drug dealing as a way of life and also opened the market to newcomers to serve neglected consumers or to those who maintained bridging ties to a potential market. The study noted that labeling theory has emphasized the way sanctions might increase involvement in criminal activities, while deterrence theory emphasizes the way sanctions might decrease this activity. They conclude, "What our findings suggest is that both may occur at the same time" (Ekland-Olson *et al.*, 1984, p. 173).

The current state of labeling theory has advanced beyond the simple idea that stigmatized persons adopt social roles and develop self-conceptions consistent with what they are socially defined as being. To varying degrees, such self-fulfilling prophesies come true depending on the social circumstances and resources available to those labeled. But more recent research makes it clear that interpersonal networks of relationships may provide a cushioning support for legitimate and nonstigmatized identities, which reduces the loss of opportunity and maintains avenues for reintegration into conventional, law-abiding pursuits. Those labeled can also collaborate in this process by selectively attributing significance and credibility to those offering support for preferred identities. When such resources for adaptation are aligned with the deterrent effect of the labeling process, it becomes possible to envision sentencing policies that increase the likelihood of diversion from a criminal to a law-abiding way of life. But research also shows that this approach will not work for all offenders. For some, the labeling process has an alienating effect that drives them deeper into identification and involvement with delinquent or criminal subcultures. For such persons, the effect of criminal sanctions may lie in the threat of disruption of the network of relationships necessary to carry out criminal enterprises successfully. The sanctions may not deter completely, but may have a "restrictive deterrence" effect in forcing a reduction of the scope and amount of criminal activity (Gibbs, 1975).

The task for the future is to develop policies that will maximize the productivity of the labeling and deterrent use of sanctions, while avoiding the harm caused by cutting off access to law-abiding paths of reintegration. To do this requires more detailed knowledge of the effect of sanctions on different types of offenders with different resource networks. Furthermore, it is not enough to show intermediate effects on attitudes, beliefs, and self-concepts. It is also necessary to link these with longer-term effects on the nature and amount of future criminal or law-abiding activity. We are now at the point where the acquisition of such knowledge could profit most from the design of experiments to test policy alternatives coupled with longitudinal follow-up to study both process and outcome. We will return to these issues in Chapter 8.

6
Restructuring the Juvenile Court

One of the most striking features of criminal justice reform over the past two decades has been the relative speed with which procedural and organizational changes in the juvenile court have taken place. The net effect has been to render juvenile court operations much more comparable to those of adult courts in their procedural requirements, operational goals and philosophies, and legislated constraints on judicial discretion. These changes in the juvenile court system have to some extent reflected the recent trend in adult court reforms away from indeterminate sentencing practices designed to facilitate rehabilitation of offenders toward determinate sentencing arrangements designed to increase equity or fairness in sentencing and the predictability of punishments. But the changes in the juvenile court go deeper than this. They reflect a sweeping repudiation of the original premises and practices of the juvenile court movement capped by proposals for the elimination of a separate juvenile court.

As one might expect, such a major policy shift in the official response to youth crime and status offenses has left a residue of unresolved philosophical and policy issues. Though it is not possible here to review these issues in a comprehensive fashion, we will illustrate the problems raised with reference to several issues now prominent in policy debates: What should be the guiding philosophy of the juvenile court? Should an increased number of serious juvenile offenders be waived or transferred to adult court jurisdiction? To what extent should the confidentiality of juvenile records be abridged by making these records available for adult court proceedings? To what extent is it desirable to divert status offenders from delinquency proceedings in juvenile courts?

The Philosophy of the Juvenile Court

Perhaps the most profound challenge of all has been the attack on the basic operating premises of the juvenile court movement as it has developed throughout this century. Grounded in the broader social reforms of the Progressive era, the juvenile court was first established in Illinois in 1899 (Schlossman, 1983). It sought to deal more effectively than the existing adult court with the problems created for children and youth, especially among immigrant families, by the increasing urbanization and industrialization of American society. It sought to employ the insights of the emerging social sciences to respond to the underlying needs and adjustment problems of children and youth rather than just the nature of their offense and prior record. The court invoked the doctrine of "parens patriae" to justify this assumption of an essentially parental role by the state. Treatment, guidance, understanding, and rehabilitation were to replace punishments because they might more effectively divert youth from a life of crime toward law-abiding pursuits.

To achieve these ends, the court introduced very informal procedures at all stages of intake, adjudication, and disposition because the object was not only to determine what the child had done and the appropriate penalty but also why and what now might best be done to correct the cause. To prevent contamination by older criminals, youth were to be detained and treated, when necessary, in separate facilities from adults. To provide the essential background information on the youthful offenders and to supervise their postadjudication treatment, probation officers were introduced to serve the court. To further distance the juvenile court approach from the criminal court, the juvenile proceedings were defined as civil rather than criminal and therefore less stigmatizing in intent.

In the 1960s and 1970s, a series of converging events provided the grounds for challenging this model of juvenile court operations. The powerful civil rights movement of the 1960s focused renewed attention on the treatment of minority groups and violation of constitutionally guaranteed protections. A series of U.S. Supreme Court decisions in the 1960s and 1970s attacked the lack of due process protections for youth implicit in the informality of juvenile court procedures. In effect, these decisions extended to juveniles most of the due process protections established for adults in criminal proceedings. The court reasoned that a process that could result in the denial of liberty and the imposition of painful punishments, such as confinement in a juvenile prison, required access to these protections.

Perhaps the most influential decision in setting this trend was *in re Gault*, 387 U.S.1 (1967), which was decided at the same time a report on juvenile delinquency was released by the President's Commission on Law Enforcement and Administration of Justice (1967). The Commission's recommendations anticipated the essential features of the Court decision that asserted for juveniles the right to receive notice of charges against them, to have legal representation, to be able to confront and cross-examine witnesses, to avoid self-incrimination, to obtain a court transcript of the hearing, and to be able to appeal the court decision. A year earlier in *Kent v. United States*, 383 U.S. 541 (1966), the Court served notice of its intention to take seriously the necessity to extend to children the constitutional protections guaranteed for adults in the criminal process. "There is evidence, in fact, that there may be grounds for concern that the child receives the worst of both worlds: that he gets neither the protections accorded to adults nor the solicitous care and regenerate treatment postulated for children" (*Kent v. United States*, 556, 1966). These actions served to question whether the informality of juvenile court proceedings could in fact serve the "best interest of the child" in the absence of the due process guarantees provided for adults charged with criminal acts.

Further challenge to the juvenile court philosophy came from the disappointing results of research on the effectiveness of rehabilitation programs. As pointed out in Chapter 3, an extensive review of these results concluded in the 1970s that virtually nothing works (Martinson, 1974). Subsequent reexamination of the evidence by the National Academy of Sciences reached similar though less pessimistic conclusions (Sechrest, White, and Brown, 1979). Such findings struck directly at the optimistic view of the juvenile court movement that referrals of youth to professionally operated treatment programs based on the insights of the behavioral sciences could succeed in diverting youth from further delinquent acts.

This questioning of the basic premises of juvenile court philosophy occurred at a time when the trend in juvenile arrests was heading for a peak in 1974 (Krisberg and Schwartz, 1983, p. 351). Public concern about youth violence and the apparent ineffectiveness of the juvenile justice response to it was reflected in steadily increasing criticism of the "permissiveness" of the courts and demands for more punitive, deterrent, and incapacitating dispositions of juveniles responsible for assaultive or repeated offenses. These reactions were part of a more general law and order trend in public opinion that demanded less concern for offenders and more for the plight of victims and for community safety.

As a result of all these developments, the juvenile court movement is now in a state of uncertainty as to its guiding philosophy. Torn between its traditional concern for meeting the needs of youth in trouble through constructive forms of treatment and the public demand for better community protection, judges are searching for a more optimum balance in sentencing between the deterrent effect of more punitive sanctions and the problem solving capacity of specific treatment, community service, or restitution measures. Many are convinced that treatment alternatives to confinement are successful for many types of young offenders. Recent evaluations of rehabilitation research are more optimistic in this regard but stress the lack of adequate data (Sechrest *et al.*, 1979). They criticize inadequacies in the rigorousness of research designs, the failure to develop a more informative array of outcome measures, and serious deficiencies in the documentation of the treatment interventions actually implemented. There is also considerable uncertainty as to the actual deterrent effect of greater use of confinement. The juvenile offender population presents a vast variety of different problems. There is a need for better data to sort out what works for different types of offenders and what sanctions tend to aggravate the threat to community safety.

Waiver to Adult Court

The delinquency cases that seem to cause the juvenile court the most troublesome public and professional criticism are the acts of violence against persons or the repeated offenses against property. The juvenile court's guiding philosophy of rehabilitation is perceived as creating a bias of leniency toward the offender at the expense of public protection and victim satisfaction. Consequently, faced with violent acts or high rates of chronic offending, critics look toward the adult criminal court for the fulfillment of retributive, deterrent, or incapacitative dispositions. The assumption is that the adult court will be more inclined to use its greater capacity for longer sentences under maximum security conditions of confinement to provide a greater measure of public protection. What evidence is available tends to create doubt about the validity of this assumption, however.

Recent studies of the decision to waive or transfer cases from the juvenile to the adult courts suggest that the initial responses of the adult court are likely to be *less* severe than the dispositions by the juvenile courts would have been in those cases. A study using the F.B.I. Uniform Crime Report data on arrests and self-report data from the 1972 National Survey of Youth concluded that youth under age 17 were more likely to be treated leniently by the adult court compared to their age mates receiving juvenile court dispositions (Ruhland *et al.*, 1982). In addition, the most recent national study reports as follows:

Our research to date revealed that adult courts in 1978 ordered fines and probation in half the cases initiated against youth through judicial waiver or prosecutorial mechanisms. Further, where confinements were ordered, maximum sentences did not exceed one year in over 40 percent of the cases. All of these sanctions are normally within juvenile court dispositional powers. (Hamparian, Estep, Muntean, Priestino, Swisher, Wallace, and White, 1982, p. 228)

Analysis of the use of waivers and their impact is complicated by the variations among the different states. The national survey found, for example, that every state (as well as the District of Columbia and the federal districts) had a judicial waiver provision in 1978 except Arkansas, Nebraska, New York, and Vermont. Thirteen states showed concurrent jurisdiction between juvenile and adult courts for some offenses, and 31 jurisdictions had statutory provisions excluding certain offenses from juvenile court jurisdiction. A total of 12 states included either 16- or 17-year-olds or just 17-year-olds within the minimum age of adult court jurisdiction. These differences had significant effects on the number referred to adult court. Though the reported cases in many jurisdictions were probably an undercount.

In 1978, the base year for data collection, the Academy determined that there were over 9,000 juveniles judicially waived to adult courts, over 2,000 youth prosecuted for serious offenses in adult courts due to concurrent jurisdiction provisions, over 1,300 youth prosecuted as adults because of excluded offense provisions, and a quarter-of-a-million 16 and 17 year olds arrested and referred to adult courts due to lower ages of jurisdiction in 12 states. The majority of youth referred to adult courts were 17 years of age, male, and white. (Hamparian *et al.*, 1982, p. 204)

As one might expect, the use of waiver varied depending on the division of jurisdiction that prevailed in a given state as well as on different philosophies and traditions. For example, waivers were more frequent in those states that retained juvenile jurisdiction over 16- and 17-year-old youth. However, most youth referred to adult court were not charged with offenses against persons, except in the states with "excluded offense" provisions. Violent offenses accounted for less than one-fourth of the judicial and prosecutorial referrals and almost one-twentieth of the arrests of 16- and 17-year-old youth in the 12 age-of-jurisdiction states.

What the survey reveals more than anything else is how little we actually know about the relative merits of transferring cases from juvenile to adult court with the expectation of more severe sentencing policies. Faced with the full range of adult criminality, the offenses of the young may appear less threatening and invite a more lenient response from the adult court judge. This also appears to be the case in England. Up to and including 1982, magistrates in England could not give a borstal sentence, involving an indeterminant custodial sentence of 6 months minimum and 24 months maximum, but had to remand to the Crown Court with a recommendation for borstal. In 1982, for persons aged 15 to 21 convicted of indictable offenses and remanded to the Crown Court for borstal, 65% received a borstal sentence, 11% received a 3-month sentence to a detention center, 2% were sentenced to prison for less than 6 months, and 1% for more than 6 months. The remaining 21% received noncustodial sentences, mostly to probation supervision or community service. This shows the greater reluctance of the Crown Court judges to impose the more severe borstal sentence in many of those remanded cases (Home Office, 1983). It is not at all certain that we gain increased deterrence, retribution, or incapacitation in this way. Youth committed by the adult court to adult prisons might become hardened and more, rather than less, likely to offend again on release. What is needed is much more careful research following comparable samples of offenders through these different experiences to provide better understanding and confident policies about the division of jurisdiction between the two courts, the relative effectiveness of the dispositional options they provide, and the efficiency of the criteria used to select offenders for differential processing and disposition.

Finally, it is not clear that legislative specification of the criteria for transfer to the adult court is adequate to secure the desired effect without a careful articulation of the underlying principles or theories of justice on which the selected criteria were chosen. For example, Barry Feld has recommended criteria based on offense and criminal record as a basis for waiver decisions in Minnesota and a recent study has reviewed the effect of legislative adoption of these criteria in that state (Feld, 1981). The study compared waivers before and after passage of the new law in 1980. The legislation was accompanied by an increase in waivers to the adult court, but the presumptive, objective criteria were ignored nearly as much as followed. Both before and after the new criteria (based on a combination of offense type and criminal record) went into effect, more youth were transferred who did not meet the criteria than those who did. In general, however, those selected showed more serious offenses and criminal histories on the average. The study concluded:

Contrary to the claims of its supporters, the objective criteria adopted by the Minnesota legislature have not proven to be an adequate means for selecting juveniles for transfer to adult court. The criteria single out many juveniles whose records do not appear to be very serious and fail to identify many juveniles whose records are characterized by violent, frequent, and persistent delinquent activity. Despite its defects and potential for abuse, the traditional discretionary process used by prosecutors and juvenile court judges to make waiver decisions appears to be more successful than the objective criteria alone in identifying the more serious juvenile offenders. Although critics of the discretionary waiver process contend that waiver decisions should be based only on objective variables related to the juvenile's behavior, the present study suggests that objective formulas—even those as sophisticated and balanced as Minnesota's—are too simplistic and too rigid to summarize such behavioral data in a reliable and consistent manner. (Osbun and Rode, 1984, pp. 199–200)

It remains to be seen just how successful more careful study of juvenile and adult careers in crime can be in identifying new criteria or offender profiles on which waiver decisions can be approved or rejected.

Confidentiality of Juvenile Records

As we indicated in our discussion of labeling theory in Chapter 5, provisions for ensuring the confidentiality of juvenile records rests on the assumption of a long-term stigmatizing effect that could foreclose future opportunities for those who wish to terminate their criminal activities and pursue law-abiding careers. It is a policy that takes account of the impulsiveness of many acts of youthful indiscretion and offers a fresh chance to begin anew. However, the increasing focus of criminal justice policy on the control of violent and chronic offenders has resulted in a growing demand for access to juvenile records for the processing of adult offenders (Boland and Wilson, 1978; Langan and Farrington, 1983; Feld, 1981). The argument holds that the confidentiality of juvenile records permits some serious offenders to appear in adult court as first-time offenders despite the existence of a serious juvenile record. This lack of coordination is seen as an artefact of the separate court jurisdictions that serious offenders can exploit to escape the control and punishment their chronic or violent offenses properly deserve. Boland and Wilson (1978) have referred to this system as "two-track justice" and regard the access to juvenile records as essential to effective crime control.

It would seem reasonable that a criminal court judge, having found a young adult guilty of a felony, should have knowledge of the offender's juvenile record in order to make an appropriate disposition. Such access is possible already in some states. According to a recent Rand inquiry in three jurisdictions (Greenwood, Petersilia, and Zimring, 1980), it appears to ensure a more severe or lenient disposition depending on the nature of the record. In many jurisdictions, the records are maintained so haphazardly as to be of little value unless better recording is provided. In reviewing the evidence in the United States on the effects of a "two-track system" of justice, Langan and Farrington concluded that little evidence existed to demonstrate greater leniency on first adult appearance when knowledge of the juvenile record was absent. In examining the English system of "one-track" justice, in which juvenile records are regularly available, they did discover that the court sentenced more severely when a juvenile record was found to exist. These findings led the investigators to conclude that more American research is needed "on sentencing inequities caused by the two-track system, and on offending rates and incarceration rates at different ages" including "more careful control of extraneous variables than is provided by legal categories alone" (Langan and Farrington, 1983, p. 546). Still another critical policy issue is how far the confidentiality of the juvenile records can be breached before the presumed benefits are lost. As youth reach the age of adult court jurisdiction, they may become increasingly sensitive to the fact that adult court records are not held in confidence and may continue to affect available opportunities for many years to come. Fear of a permanent record may lead some to abandon crime providing the juvenile record remains confidential or sealed. This deterrent effect may be lost if juvenile records become readily accessible. The transitional age between juvenile and adult legal status is one involving many critical career decisions with respect to marriage, family, occupation, friends, and life-style as well as criminal activity. We need to know more about the significance of juvenile record availability in the matrix of these decisions. This means exploring on a longitudinal basis the significance of confidentiality as a protection against labeling effects or an invitation to crime while still a juvenile, and the possible loss of the deterrent effect of an adult record when the confidentiality of the juvenile record is sacrificed.

Decriminalizing Status Offenses

Another major consequence of the changing philosophy of the juvenile court, rivaling the movement to formalize juvenile court procedures, has been the movement to divert status offenders from the delinquency adjudication process. The traditional philosophy of the juvenile court posed no problem for the inclusion of truants, runaways, curfew violators, or drug-abusing youth within the scope of the delinquency petition. The benign conception of the court as a substitute parent concerned more with the underlying adjustment problems of the child rather than with the nature of the offense appeared to justify this inclusion. Status offenders were often also involved in minor delinquent acts or perceived as especially vulnerable and at high risk of such involvement unless these problems could be promptly addressed. Parents, school authorities, police, and social agency workers welcomed the involvement of the court as a last resort to save the child from the consequences of ungovernability. Girls especially were seen as requiring such control and treatment to protect them from sexual exploitation as juveniles. Status offenders were confined and treated in the same programs as delinquents. With the decline of the rehabilitative ideal and the advent of the due process revolution in delinquency proceedings, it no longer appeared justifiable to include status offenders in the same process as those whose delinquent acts were also crimes for adults.

These developments raised a number of policy issues that have not been wholly resolved. At this point we wish to consider two major issues that are of central importance in arriving at an effective and constructive policy for status offenders. Should the court retain jurisdiction over such cases in some fashion or be divested of this authority? If the court retained jurisdiction, should it be prohibited from confining status offenders in residential institutions with or without committed delinquents?

Many states have elected to retain control over status offenders by creating an alternative petition route in juvenile court variously designated as persons, children, or minors in need of services (labeled respectively, Pins, Chins, or Mins). At least two states, Maine and Washington, have opted to divest the court of authority to dispose of status offender cases. The implementation of this policy in the state of Washington has recently been studied and reported by Ann Schneider (1984). Full divestiture prohibits the court from imposing any official requirement and makes referral to other service agencies voluntary. The state of Washington legislature moved to reduce the use of coercion in status offense cases throughout the 1970s and consolidated its approach in an extensive set of amendments in 1979. The study revealed that coercive control over status offenders "was virtually eliminated by the divestiture law" in the two cities studied, Seattle and Yakima. Some compromise control measures proved necessary, however, and other problems developed. Police were permitted to bring endangered status offenders and runaways to a crisis residential center operated by the state's Department of Social and Health Services. The crisis center was then authorized to refer such offenders to detention for up to 24 hours under defined circumstances. However, "by 1980, the number admitted to detention had dropped to zero, statewide." No evidence could be found of a net-widening effect of the divestiture law in the sense of expanding social service control over more children than would have been processed by the court system. However, there was evidence of relabeling to permit processing as a delinquent offender and a tendency to sentence more harshly those delinquents with a prior history of status-type behavior. Schneider concludes that these discretionary reactions were used "to bring status offenders under the jurisdiction of the court at a rate almost as great as had existed prior to the reform" (1984, pp. 347–376). Although "pure" status offenders (those not also involved in delinquency) were removed from court authority, the inability to conduct follow-up studies of the subsequent adjustment of the youth makes it difficult to decide whether divestiture is a successful crime reduction or treatment policy.

Another avenue for mitigating the potentially harmful effects of court dispositions on the treatment of status offenders is to prohibit their commitment to training schools for delinquents. The objectives of such policies are to eliminate the stigmatizing effect of this type of confinement and to avoid exposure to criminalizing influences with the formation of new delinquent peer associations. This type of recommendation was urged by the national crime commissions of the 1960s and 1970s and was a major thrust of the 1974 Juvenile Justice and Delinquency Prevention Act, which established the Office of Juvenile Justice and Delinquency Prevention in the U.S. Department of Justice. An extensive report on the implementation of this policy was conducted by the Panel on the Deinstitutionalization of Children and Youth of the National Research Council (Handler and Zatz, 1982). It found wide variations among the states in the degree of commitment to this policy and its implementation. In general, however, it found substantial reductions in the use of institutional confinement for status offenders, a conclusion that independent analysis by Krisberg and Schwartz (1983) has confirmed more recently. However, here again there are major reservations about the total effect similar to those noted above relating to divestiture. Kobrin and Klein (1983) discovered an unintended net-widening effect in which the creation of community alternatives instead of institutional confinement resulted in more youth becoming subject to official control as status offenders. There is evident also a relabeling process in which status offenders committing incidental acts of delinquency are charged as delinquents (Klein, 1979).

Despite the net-widening and relabeling effects, the National Research Council's panel found considerable concern among social service professionals that the problems of many runaway, truant, and ungovernable children were simply being ignored until more serious misconduct occurred. The most important reservation of the panel, however, was the limited scope of the study, which did not allow for follow-up assessments of the longer run impact of the deinstitutionalization policy on the lives of the youth and their families. This is a complaint voiced as well by other investigators who have become concerned, as was the panel, about the possible reinstitutionalization of youth within a "hidden" system of juvenile control operated by mental health, welfare, or chemical dependency program staff (Schwartz, Jackson-Beeck, and Anderson, 1984). There is clearly a need for longer-term studies to determine whether diversion from institutions to alternative community services has been beneficial or not before more definitive judgments about these policies can be reached.

Conclusions

From the foregoing it is apparent that the juvenile court philosophy, its use of waivers to adult court, the confidentiality of its records, and its jurisdiction over status offenders are all undergoing critical reexamination and change. It is also clear that many of the criticisms and alternative policy proposals arise in large part from a major shift in conceptualizing the appropriate jurisdiction, procedures, dispositional alternatives, and objectives of the juvenile court. The juvenile court is under pressure to surrender jurisdiction over its serious chronic and violent offenders on the one hand and its noncriminal and minor offenders on the other. Coupled with the increasing formalization of the court, these trends threaten the existence of the juvenile court as a separate institution. It is noteworthy that the U.S. Supreme Court in its *McKeiver v. Pennsylvania* (1971) decision expressed a reluctance to permit the assertion of due process guarantees to herald the end of the juvenile court movement.

It appears that the due process revolution in the juvenile court has proceeded under the assumption that equal protection before the law should be provided as much for juveniles as for adults. As the model of adult court protections is applied to the juvenile court, the two courts come to resemble one another more exactly and raise doubts as to the necessity of a separate juvenile court. Before such a conclusion could be reached, however, it would be necessary to examine the organization and practices of the juvenile court in relation to its network of services. The juvenile court plays a central role in mobilizing essential services in individual cases and in supporting the growth of more effective placement options for delinquent youth. The obligation of the court to provide due process in delinquency proceedings is only part of its institutional obligation and capability. It must also develop some measure of competence in dealing with the network of services concerned with helping youth solve problems of growth and development. The obligation to provide a just process of adjudication is matched by the obligation to provide effective and appropriate dispositions. The juvenile court movement was motivated in considerable part by the idea that a specialized court for juveniles could best develop this dispositional competence. Future research must, therefore, address this set of obligations, as well, before elimination of the juvenile court for delinquency proceedings can be considered as a justifiable policy.

7
The Effects of Imprisonment

Except for the death penalty, imprisonment is the severest sanction available to the United States courts in sentencing convicted criminals. In recent years there has been a substantial increase in the number of offenders confined in prison. The resulting overcrowding has created serious management problems, federal court intervention concerning the conditions of confinement, and strong pressure to build new institutions despite the high costs involved. It is therefore timely to consider two major policy issues: How effective is the use of imprisonment in achieving the goals of criminal justice policy? What do we need to know about imprisonment to increase its utility as an instrument of crime control?

Before proceeding to a discussion of these issues, a few figures on increases in prison population, housing capacity, and costs may help to underscore the urgency of the problem. It is commonly noted that criminal justice policies in the 1970s and 1980s have resulted in a greater use of imprisonment. As shown in Table 7.1, the number of persons serving time in federal and state prisons has more than doubled in the past decade with the largest percentage increases in population occurring in 1981 and 1982 at 12% and falling off to 6% in 1983 and 1984. Similarly, the rate of imprisonment increased steadily from 104 per 100,000 population in 1974 to 188 in 1984.

With such sizable increases in population, it is not surprising to find the prisons in most states are strained beyond their rated capacity. A recent report by the U.S. Bureau of Justice Statistics summarizes the situation confronting prison administrators struggling with the shortage of housing in 1983 as follows:

* The entire prison system in seven states (and all male penal facilities in one additional state) were operating under court order to reduce overcrowded conditions;
* 24 jurisdictions were operating one or more facilities under court order or consent decree, and 9 others had litigation pending;
* 18 states reported a total of nearly 8,100 sentenced prisoners held in local jails because of crowding in State prisons;
* 15 states reported a total of 21,420 prisoners who received early releases during 1983 because of crowding in State prisons;
* State and Federal prison systems reported that, on the average, they were operating at about 110% capacity;

* 1 in every 10 inmates was estimated to reside in a prison built before 1875 and the average inmate resided in a prison nearly 40 years old. [Bureau of Justice Statistics Bulletin (BJSB, 1984b, p. 8]

Thus, in addition to crowding prisoners into cells, dormitories, hospitals, and other utilizable bed space, administrators have arranged housing for state prisoners in local jails and have experimented with varous early release mechanisms. A further option, of course, is to add new facilities to accommodate the increased demand for prison space. Nearly 42,000 beds were added as a result of facility renovation or construction in 1981 and 1982 (BJSB, 1984b, p. 5). Furthermore, the 51 jurisdictions reported more than 28,000 beds under construction in 1982 while 49 of these jurisdictions reported an additional 73,600 beds planned (BJSB, 1984b). A survey of average construction costs in 1982 dollars ranged from a low of $34,000 to a high of $110,000 per prison bed, depending on the security level required, siting costs, space allowances, financing, regional variation in construction costs, etc. (BJSB, 1983, p. 93). Capital expenditures increased throughout the 1970s to a peak of $760 million in 1981 (BJSB, 1984b, p. 6). In addition, capital improvements based on bond issues or other special revenue mechanisms grew to $1.3 billion in 1983 (BJSB, 1984b, p. 6). Imprisonment, of course, is also the most expensive sentencing option available to the court and led to direct operational costs in 1983 of over $5.5 billion for state correctional systems, an increase of 393% over the $1.4 billion reported for 1973 (BJSB, 1984b, p. 6). Estimates of the average annual cost in 1982 for one adult offender in a state prison ranged from $5,000 to $23,000 (BJSB, 1983, p. 92). About twice as much is spent per capita by local and state government for police protection as compared to corrections. However, from 1971 to 1979, per capita

TABLE 7.1. Changes in total state and federal prison population, 1974–84.

Year	Number	Change (%)	Rate per 100,000 population
1974	229,721		104
1975	253,816	10.5	113
1976	278,000	9.5	123
1977 (custody)	291,667	4.9	129
1977 (jurisdiction)	300,024		
1978	307,276	2.4	135
1979	314,457	2.3	136
1980	329,821	4.9	139
1981	369,930	12.2	153
1982	413,806	11.9	170
1983	437,248	5.7	179
1984	463,866	6.1	188

Note. Before 1977, National Prisoner Statistics reports were based on custody population; beginning in 1977, they were based on the jurisdiction population. Both are shown for 1977 to facilitate year-to-year comparison.
Source. "Prisoners in 1984," *Bureau of Justice Statistics Bulletin*, April, 1985, pp. 1–2; and *Sourcebook of Criminal Justice Satistics, 1984*, p. 648 (Bureau of Justice Statistics, U.S. Department of Justice, Washington, DC).

correctional expenditures by state and local governments increased by 29% compared to 10% for the police and 40% for the courts, prosecution, and public defense (BJSB, 1983, p. 101).

Clearly, substantial increases in the rate of imprisonment such as we have experienced in recent years is a costly policy decision in dollars alone, without regard to the human costs for staff and prisoners alike of operating and surviving in dangerously overcrowded and federally adjudicated unconstitutional conditions. It is, thus, especially important to examine what we know and do not know about the assumptions on which such policies are based.

Evidence for Assumptions in Imprisonment Policies

The increased use of imprisonment as a sanction for crime has been accompanied by a relatively intense reexamination and debate about the justifications for its use. Utilitarian justifications seek to advance the goal of crime control through various means, such as rehabilitation programs, the deterrent effect of imprisonment itself, the public reassertion of the moral validity of the violated laws, or the removal of criminal opportunities through the incapacitative effect of imprisonment. The retributive justification for imprisonment seeks to administer justice by exacting a measure of pain in proportion to the harm inflicted by the crime. The appeal of imprisonment as a penal sanction, and undoubtedly its durability, may lie in its apparent ability to fulfill all of these justifications at the same time. The important question to address, however, is how adequately these justifications are supported by the evidence on the effects of imprisonment.

Rehabilitation of Offenders

Perhaps more studies have been directed toward determining the effect of prison rehabilitation programs than any of the other justifications for imprisonment. The accumulated empirical evaluations of these programs have proved disappointing for advocates of rehabilitation. As mentioned earlier, the widely circulated assessment by Martinson and his colleagues has been verified in large measure by a subsequent Panel on Research on Rehabilitation Techniques organized by the National Research Council of the National Academy of Sciences (Lipton et al., 1975; Sechrest et al., 1979; Martin et al., 1981). The panel drew the following conclusions.

The current state of knowledge about rehabilitation of criminal offenders is cause for grave concern, particularly in view of the obvious importance of the problem. After 40 years of research and literally hundreds of studies, almost all the conclusions that can be reached have to be formulated in terms of what we do not know. The one positive conclusion is discouraging: the research methodology that has been brought to bear on the problem of finding ways to rehabilitate criminal offenders has been generally so inadequate that only a relatively few studies warrant any unequivocal interpretations. The entire body of research appears to justify only the conclusion that we do not know of any program or method of rehabilitation that could be guaranteed to reduce the criminal activity of released offenders. Although a generous reviewer of the literature might discern some glimmers of hope, those glimmers are so few, so scattered, and so inconsistent that they do not serve as a basis for any recommendation other than continued research.

Furthermore, a more penetrating inquiry into the nature of the problem of rehabilitation and the programs and methods that have been tried leads to the conclusion that there is even less in the research than meets the eye. The techniques that have been tested seem rarely to have been devised to be strong enough to offer realistic hope that they would rehabilitate offenders, especially imprisoned felons. In general, techniques have been tested as isolated treatments rather than as complex combinations, which would seem more suited to the task. And even when techniques have been tested in good designs, insufficient attention has been paid to maintaining their integrity, so that often the treatment to be tested was delivered in a substantially weakened form. It is also not clear that all the theoretical power and the individual imagination that could be invoked in the planning of rehabilitative efforts have ever been capitalized on. Thus, the recommendation in this report that has the strongest support is that more and better thinking and research should be invested in efforts to devise programs for offender rehabilitation. (Sechrest et al., 1979, pp. 3–4)

The panel felt that some treatments might work well with "certain subgroups of offenders" and offered some suggestions for programs that might be tried.

Among the logical possibilities for innovative rehabilitation efforts, several seem especially worthy of consideration for development and evaluation: extensive family interventions; intervention efforts directed at the offender very early in his criminal career...; restitution by the offender; increased support...after the prisoner's release from prison rather than before release; employment and vocational programs; and alternative sentencing and confinement. Although some of these interventions may be costly, it may be worth a great deal to show in principle that rehabilitation can work. (Sechrest et al., 1979, pp. 8–9).

In conclusion, the panel called on "appropriate funding agencies [to] support research on criminal rehabilitation, while making the criteria for funding more rigorous with respect to experimental design, theoretical rationale, and monitoring of integrity and strength of treatment" (Sechrest et al., 1979, p. 10).

Faced with such discouraging assessments, many policy analysts urged abandonment of rehabilitation as an organizing objective of the prison system. In most maximum security prisons, of course, the small number of programs designed to deal with the rehabilitative needs of the inmates served often as show-piece programs that cast a rhetorical gloss of rehabilitation over a basically punitive custodial system. A recent survey of correctional administrators by the National Institute of Corrections, however, indicates that the vast majority are not prepared to give up rehabilitative programs altogether (Smith, 1983). They appear convinced that such programs will work for subgroups of offenders with both the need and motivation to take advantage of them. Furthermore, such programs offer some relief from the personally destructive features of prison life: the debilitating idleness; loss of autonomy and ability to exercise initiative; the latent and overt threats of force and violence; and the routinization, monotony, and regimentation of activities and relationships.

The efforts to create academic and vocational training opportunities, self-help programs for drug abusers, individual and group therapy and counseling possibilities, and paid work in prison industries also serve an important symbolic function. They express confidence and hope in the ability of people to change when they become motivated to seek new directions in their lives. They embody a continuing faith that such directions are never fully determined by the past. Prison administrators now appear more inclined to make participation in such programs voluntary rather than coerced as a condition for release on parole. It appears that in the prison world, the rehabilitative ideal is not dead so much as reduced in expectation to accord more fully with the realities and limitations of the prison experience (Morris, 1974).

In concluding his insightful analysis of the current decline of the rehabilitative ideal and its future role, Francis Allen underscores the state's obligation as follows:

> . . . the central justification [for providing facilitative rehabilitation programs] rests on a proposition of public morality. In dealing even with those who have seriously breached community norms of conduct, it is wrong for the state to strip all hope and opportunity for self-development from the human beings within its custody and care; it is accordingly part of the state's obligation to facilitate, where feasible, prisoners' aspirations for knowledge and growth. (1981, p. 84)

We are left then with many questions about such programs: What types of programs are likely to be most successful? What types of inmates respond effectively to the different types of programs that can be made available? What types of measures reveal best the changes attributable to the programs? What effect do such changes have on recidivism rates or other indicators of postprison adjustment? What kinds of continuing support during the postrelease period are needed to sustain the changes achieved and their effect on future criminality? What types of research procedures must be instituted to determine what works and what does not?

General and Individual Deterrence

When the legislature wishes to raise the level of the publicly perceived moral culpability of an offense, it will frequently attach to its denunciation of the act a new option of imprisonment as a sanction or extend the maximum allowable sentence to prison. Currently the attack on drunken driving provides an illustration. Use of the threat of confinement in this way is premised on the assumption that the social disgrace and deprivations of imprisonment have a powerful general deterrent effect on potential offenders. It is also assumed that the experience of imprisonment will help to deter the individual offender from repeating his offense in order to escape further confinement.

Considering the pervasiveness of these deterrent assumptions embedded in the criminal law, it is remarkable how little evidence can be assembled to document these assumed effects. Perhaps the most illuminating exploration of these matters has been undertaken by Johannes Andenaes of the law faculty of the University of Oslo. However, of his work and that of others he notes that

Much has been written about general prevention; much talented effort has been spent in exploring its operation and importance. But the empirical data are still lacking. If any attempt has been made to include it at all, it has usually—as in this paper—occurred by the use of chance observations, plus ordinary psychological theories. I believe we can make some progress in this way. But we shall not have firm ground to stand on before a systematic investigation is made into the effect of penal law and its enforcement on the citizen's behavior, and into the interrelation between the legal system and the other factors which govern behavior. (Andenaes, 1977, pp. 37–38)

General deterrence seeks to prevent criminal conduct through the fear of punishment. It also peforms an educative or moralizing function for the public by denouncing those acts that are proscribed by the criminal law. To the extent that these proscriptions are assimilated into fairly stable attitudes against engaging in such conduct, the moralizing effect of the criminal law may deter even where the probability of punishment is low. In general, however, effective deterrence is linked to a public perception of the certainty of enforcement. For example, as mentioned in Chapter 3, the publicity attending stricter penalties against drunken driving produced an initial public compliance that tended to dissipate as the public discovered that the level of enforcement or its certainty was much less than anticipated (Ross, 1973). Apparently an unenforced threat lacks the credibility to deter. The sharp increase in the crime rate as a consequence of police strikes or other breakdowns in the enforcement system are often pointed to as further evidence of the general deterrent effect of the criminal justice system.

It is important to note at the outset that the maintenance of a free, yet orderly, society rests more securely on the internalization of moral standards and defenses against crime than on externally enforced sanctions. Most citizens do not need the deterrent effect of such sanctions, except perhaps as a symbolic reassertion of the validity of the moral prohibitions that they share (Walker, 1980). In fact, surveys of the public show that most people have only a hazy idea about the sanctions provided by the criminal law or the probability of apprehension and punishment. The general tendency is to exaggerate the certainty of discovery and the severity of punishment. However, the case for general deterrence relies more on the common sense observations of everyday life than on systematic empirical data or analysis. The restraint of impulses to engage in forbidden conduct because of fear of undesirable and painful consequences is a familiar experience for most people. It is on such common reactions that support for the deterrent effect of punishment rests. But we need better understanding of how well this process works to deter potential offenders from crime. The widespread prevalence of acts of law violation revealed by self-report studies suggests the presence of ample motivations to crime that fear of punishment and loss of social reputation must somehow constrain. We need to know more about how this affects persons living under different social, economic, and cultural conditions. More specifically, we need to know how important the threat of imprisonment is in such calculations.

We are not much better off with respect to the state of the evidence on individual or special deterrence that may result from the imposition of punishment. How much does the threat of further punishment constrain the behavior of offenders already imprisoned? For most prisoners, the stake in social reputation is already lost or marginal at best and the high rates of recidivism among former prisoners suggests that fear of prison may also be much reduced. Clearly there must be a great deal of variation among different types of offenders in these respects and better understanding of the variations would make for a more accurate cost–benefit assessment of imprisonment policies. Undoubtedly part of the impetus toward more conservative sentencing policies and greater use of imprisonment rests on assumptions about general and individual deterrence, but we simply lack adequate evidence about their validity and importance for crime control (Zimring and Hawkins, 1973; Blumstein, Cohen, and Nagin, 1978).

Collective and Selective Incapacitation

Incapacitation offers the simplest justification for imprisonment inasmuch as crime in the community might be reduced by the number of crimes the confined offender would have committed if free. This possibility of reducing crimes by different types of incapacitation usually involves a strategy that would result in the same sentence for persons convicted of the same offense or who had comparable prior records. Estimtes of the amount of crime reduction vary depending on the assumptions made about the average annual crime rate for individual offenders, the probability of replacement of criminal activity by others, and the amount of crime committed by persons not apprehended. The larger the individual crime rate of sentenced offenders, the greater will be the expected incapacitation effect. Another approach uses the past criminal records of persons currently convicted of crime to explore crime reduction under different possible sentencing policies, such as a mandatory five-year term after any felony conviction as an adult or after a repeat felony conviction. The estimated effect on crime reduction is in the range of 10 to 20% (Cohen, 1983a, p. 27). Part of the reason for this limited impact is that many offenders have no prior adult convictions. The effects of such a strategy on prison populations, however, can be prohibitive, doubling or tripling the numbers in confinement.

Because prison confinement is so expensive, more recent analyses have explored the possibilities of a selective incapacitation strategy. The idea here is to select out for imprisonment the small number of very active offenders who commit a disproportionate amount of the crimes. If these offenders can be identified early enough in their crime careers, substantial reductions in crime may be achieved without greatly increasing prison populations. For example, the research results obtained by Peter Greenwood indicated that the number of robberies by adults in California could be lowered by 20% with only an increase of

2.5% in the prison population (Greenwood with Abrahamse, 1982). Obviously, if such a strategy could be made to work, it would have great appeal to states trying to reduce crime while keeping prison populations under control. This approach has been criticized, however, because of empirical problems involved in predicting future conduct and because of troublesome ethical questions (see also Chapter 2).

The major problem with current efforts to predict future criminality is that the variables used thus far produce high false-positive predictions. John Monahan's (1981) recent review of efforts to predict violence found that the best predictions produced false-positive rates over 60% of the time, indicating that two out of every three persons predicted to be violent were not, in fact, observed to be violent. However, the actual false-positive rate may be lower because many who commit offenses are not arrested. Greenwood's false-positive rate of 55% was only slightly less, and unresolved empirical issues remain in his study. A recent reanalysis of the Greenwood data noted several of these problems. Estimations by Greenwood were based on the prior crimes of known high-rate offenders and thus it is difficult to decide how well the resulting scales would work in identifying high-rate offenders *prospectively* rather than retrospectively. There are also problems of *internal* and *external validation*. Would the scale work as well if applied to a new group of imprisoned offenders with comparable high rates of past offense? More important, would it work as well if applied in court to a newly charged sample of offenders? Furthermore, in constructing the scale, reliance had to be placed on the *self-reported* crimes of offenders, a procedure that would seem unlikely to work well at the sentencing stage (Cohen, 1983b).

Ethical issues have also been raised against a selective incapacitation strategy. Some have argued that it is not fair to punish for predicted crimes that are unlikely to occur. Furthermore, it is troubling to rely on such factors as employment, education, or residential stability because these variables are highly associated with class and race and are thus likely to result in more severe punishments for minorities and the poor.

Following a careful review of the research and ethical issues, Jacqueline Cohen suggests the use of collective incapacitation policies based on criminal career data in order to avoid some of the problems raised by a selective incapacitation policy. This approach is described as follows:

The key variables include empirical estimates of average individual arrest and crime rates and the average length of criminal careers. Efforts are also made to identify variations in criminal careers associated with the nature of the current crime and with prior criminal record.

The goal is to identify classes of offenders who, on average, would remain active at high rates... Robbery and burglary defendants emerge as prime candidates for incapacitation. They commit these offenses, on average, at relatively high rates, and have relatively short careers. Short prison terms for these offenders have the potential to avert large portions of their expected careers and thereby to reduce robbery and burglary rates.

...Minimum 2-year terms imposed on all adult offenders convicted of robbery [in a District of Columbia sample of offenders] would result in an 8 percent reduction in robberies by adults, while increasing the total prison population by 7 percent. (Cohen, 1983b, p. 7)

This approach is undergoing more rigorous examination by a panel on criminal careers appointed by the National Research Council. By relying solely on present and past criminal records and uniform treatment of similar offenders, it avoids some of the ethical problems inherent in the selective incapacitation policies.

Whether the impact on prison population and the ethical and prediction problems of an incapacitation policy can be resolved acceptably remains to be seen, but there are other issues that also need further research. We need to know much more about the way the prison experience affects different types of inmates because for some it appears to increase their disposition to commit crime and to use violence to deal with personal problems; for others it signals the end of their career in crime. It is apparent that the organization of the prison environment and its programmatic opportunities affects offenders in different ways. However, much research still treats the prison experience as a black box that prisoners enter and leave without much understanding of its effects, or the research evaluates relatively limited demonstration programs. Furthermore, we do not know what the optimum sentences might be for different classes of offenders; previous research suggests that overly severe sentences are associated with higher recidivism rates. It is commonplace to note that prisons serve as schools of crime, but this is certainly not true for all offenders. If incapacitation policies are to be pursued in the future, then we need much better theories and research evidence on the nature and effect of exposure to prison life.

Retribution

The attack on the concept of rehabilitation as a justification for treatment under conditions of coercive confinement precipitated an extensive scholarly debate about the objectives of punishment. Perhaps most conspicuous in this reexamination of basic philosophical principles has been the restoration of the concept of retribution to a position of prominence. The dominance of utilitarian justifications for punishment in the 19th and 20th centuries obscured the degree to which retributive principles continued to figure in criminal justice decisions. The retributive position has an apparent clarity and simplicity that seems to accord well with common sense attitudes about punishing offenders. It posits that human actors have free will and therefore the ability to make responsible choices of possible actions to undertake or reject. To punish from a retributive position one need only look back to the harm resulting from the crime and devise a punishment proportionate to this harm. Predictions of future dangerousness are irrelevant, therefore, to this decision.

Behind this apparent simplicity, however, lurk complex assumptions. The law provides for excuses or defenses to criminal acts that turn on the issue of whether the person's condition or the situation was one in which a responsible, free choice could be made. Responsible choice also presumes the formation of a conscious

intent to commit the crime with knowledge of its forbidden character. Even when
these issues are resolved in any particular case, the question of the proportionality of the punishment to the criminal harm poses difficult problems. There exists
no agreed-upon scale of equivalences between the harm caused and the penalty
exacted. How are the deprivations and pains of imprisonment or other alternative
punishments to be made commensurate with the harm induced by the crime? The
initial results of a national survey developed and analyzed by Marvin Wolfgang
and his associates indicate that there is considerable public consensus in scoring
the relative severity of crime, but the problem of establishing the appropriate
proportion between harm and penalty remains (BJSB, 1984a). There is also the
assumption that retributive punishment should foster in the victims of crime a
sense of satisfaction that justice has been done and the prevailing order of legally
established norms restored. But the extent to which punishments achieve this is
anybody's guess in most cases.

It now seems much clearer that the system of justice in most states represents
a mixture of retributive and utilitarian motivations and practices that is much
more complex than single-minded adherence to any particular justification for
punishment. There is as little evidence that imprisonment fulfills the aims of
retribution as there is for the utilitarian objectives discussed above. Without
more extensive research it will prove difficult to devise adequate measures of the
way in which imprisonment responds to the issues of proportionality, victim
satisfaction, and effective restoration of violated norms.

Effects of the Prison Experience

One clear message that emerges from the foregoing brief review of the relation
of imprisonment to the achievement of major objectives of the criminal justice
system is the need to understand more concretely the impact of the prison
experience on those confined. What effect does this experience have on
prisoners' attitudes, values, and beliefs, on their self-image and self-esteem, and
on their capacity to avoid harm and draw benefit? What types of relationships are
available or experienced in the prison world? What happens to relationships with
the external world of family, friends, neighbors, and employers? In the final analysis, what effect does imprisonment have on the postprison experiences and conduct of the released offender? Better answers to these questions will undoubtedly
have important policy implications for the structure of sentencing decisions, the
design of more constructive environments for confinement, and the development
of programs to make imprisonment a more effective instrument of crime control.

Research on the impact of imprisonment shows that the effects vary widely
depending on the type of offender, the length of time to be served, and the type
of facility and its management practices. Variation by age, sex, racial and ethnic
identity, social background, type of offense, and prior criminal and correctional
experience can be the basis for classification into different facilities or programs.
Even within the same facility the adjustment problems encountered can vary

significantly in relation to these characteristics. Whether a person is serving a long or short term in prison also makes a significant difference in the types of problems encountered and the resources available to deal with them. Long-termers tend to seek out more stable, predictable, and safe niches or situations within the prison system (Toch, 1977).

There are also great variations in the United States in the level of threats to personal safety, integrity, and well-being that offenders experience in different states and types of facilities. Most states with large prison populations operate facilities that differ in custody and security levels. The U.S. Bureau of Justice Statistics reports that, "in 1979, 52 percent of all prison inmates were held under maximum security; 37 percent under medium security; and 11 percent under minimum security" (BJSB, 1983). About 4% of the minimum security prisoners were housed in smaller community-based units to facilitate treatment, work, school, or release arrangements. In general, the medium and minimum institutions house fewer inmates and are much more likely to have been constructed in recent years. "About 41 percent of the maximum security prisons were built before 1925; more than 87 percent of the medium-custody prisons were built after 1925; and more than 60 percent of the minimum security prisons were built after 1950" (BJSB, 1983). Since the older, larger maximum security prisons house those inmates regarded as the most violent or chronic threats to public safety, we shall focus especially on the effects of confinement in such facilities. This should not, however, divert attention from the central importance of undertaking comparative studies of the differential experiences and effects of imprisonment in facilities of varying size, security level, or available program opportunities.

Relationships Internal to the Prison

Because of the high priority accorded custody considerations in maximum security prisons, relations between prisoners and staff tend to be impersonal and given over to the communication of authoritative directives. This is, of course, much less true of the program than the custodial staff, but there are many more guards than program staff members and custody considerations take precedence when problems arise. Furthermore, the very low ratio of staff to inmates in large prisons forces a stricter pattern of regimentation and rule enforcement to maintain order and curb violence. What tends to develop is an official subculture among the staff organized around custodial problems and set in opposition to an inmate subculture which prisoners cultivate in response. This oppositional stance can lead to such alienation and hostility that an escalation of violence between staff and inmates may produce brutal and degrading conditions for both groups.

One of the central problems in prison management is to find ways to defuse this confrontation and to create new patterns of staff–inmate relationships with less harmful consequences while still maintaining essential levels of security. There is recent research evidence that replacing an autocratic system of hierarchical authority headed by the prison warden with a more decentralized, bureaucratic management system can prove beneficial (Jacobs, 1977b). What is needed here are more comparative studies of different prison systems, coupled with experimentation and long-term follow-up to determine what works best. It is clear from studies of juvenile facilities, for example, that decentralizing into smaller units with more group process and shared decision-making by staff and inmates can overcome much of the alienation in staff–inmate relationships typically encounted in larger institutions (Feld, 1977). Whether similar practices will work in prisons needs to be explored; also to be explored is how this diffusion process can be successfully instituted. Unless conditions can be created in which staff and inmates can enter into more effective communication, there is little hope of inducing constructive change in prisoners during confinement or, more modestly, of simply reducing the levels of harm and violence.

Studies of prison systems by sociologists over the past 30 years have tended to focus on descriptive accounts of the social roles available to inmates and the norms, values, and beliefs transmitted in the inmate subcultures (Thomas and Peterson, 1977). A major source of controversy has revolved around the issue of whether these features of inmate subcultures are imported from delinquent and criminal subcultures on the outside or are formed in opposition to the official culture of the prison itself (Irwin and Cressey, 1962). It now seems apparent that both processes are at work and the relative importance of each process varies among institutions (Bowker, 1977). Longitudinal surveys of prisoners, comparative studies of these institutional differences, and experimentation with measures for reducing both the importation and oppositional effects are needed to inform prison policies and practices. It is perhaps easier to devise means by which official expectations of relationships among staff, among inmates, and between staff and inmates can be changed to foster a more constructive social climate in the prison. It may be more difficult to determine how the contribution of imported criminal values to the inmate subculture can be controlled. In recent years, for example, prison officials have been confronted with the emergence of warfare among gangs of prisoners organized along racial and ethnic divisions (Jacobs, 1977b). The prison gangs have their counterparts in urban areas where conflict occurs over the control of territory or criminal enterprises such as the drug trade. In prison, the gangs are protective of their members but predatory toward other groups or unprotected individuals who may be victimized by sexual assaults, psychological or physical degradation, or theft of belongings. Unprotected individuals often feel compelled to accept homosexual liaisons and debasing relationships with gang members to achieve some protection from gang rape or other kinds of exploitation.

The increasing concentration of habitual criminal and violent offenders for longer sentences in maximum security prisons in the last decade has strained the capacity of prison administrators to create or maintain a safe and supportive environment for those confined (Irwin, 1980; Carroll, 1974). In the larger systems, transfers of troublemakers or gang leaders is possible to some extent, but such a policy may exacerbate the problem by spreading dissention to formerly peaceful institutions. This situation raises a basic policy dilemma. Is it better to spread out the more violent and exploitive inmates among different institutions in order to reduce the danger of collective violence and riots that might come from their mutual support of one another? Or is it better to concentrate them in a single facility where physical and custodial constraints can be intensified? One policy appears to invite contagion and the other homicidal assaults and riots.

Most maximum security prisons have internal segregation units for the punishment of rule violators, but these are also used for the longer-term segregation of assaultive prisoners. In addition, the prisons are increasingly called upon to provide protective custody for those unable to survive in the general population because of constant sexual assaults, default on gambling or drug trade debts, or because of prior testimony as a state's witness against former associates. Life in a protective custody unit can be a much more confining existence for those threatened than for those in the general population whom they fear. Such problems of prison management deserve much more experimentation and evaluation of alternative solutions than they now receive. The aim should be not only to test the policies but to determine what both the long- and short-term consequences may be for the prisoners affected by them.

The Impact on Prisoners

One of the key issues relating to imprisonment is the extent to which prisoners experience changes that increase or reduce the likelihood of further criminal activity following release. Those confined in prison generally experience a loss of autonomy and initiative in comparison to their former existence. It is a common complaint among prisoners that they can decide nothing for themselves and are reduced to a child-like state. The intensity of this feeling obviously will vary for different individuals depending on their own personal resources for adjusting to a monotonous, boring, authoritative, and frequently dehumanizing situation. Furthermore, maximum security facilities vary considerably in the degree to which opportunities are created that challenge the initiative and resourcefulness of the inmates. In industrial and vocational shops, schools, and small group discussion and self-study programs, prisoners may encounter more rewarding forms of self-expression and participation in decision-making. Other prisoners are able to discount the dependency implicated in relations with prison staff by finding resources for self-esteem in interactions within the inmate subcultural system of rewarded behavior. Several studies have found, for example, that the sense of powerlessness and alienation induced by the prison system led to antistaff attitudes, a negative attitude toward prison programs, and a strong identification with the inmate subculture (Smith and Hepburn, 1979).

What these types of findings suggest is the possibility of devising ways to reduce alienation and the oppositional nature of the inmate subculture by using various forms of group decision-making and counseling. Though these practices have been shown to reduce alienation in juvenile facilities, the results thus far in adult prisons appear less promising (Feld, 1977; McEwen, 1978). One of the most carefully controlled experimental studies of group counseling in a California prison found, for example, that the counseling had little effect on the endorsement of inmate norms and beliefs in opposition to staff by the experimental as compared to the control group (Kassebaum *et al.*, 1971). It may be that a positive outcome can only be achieved in smaller, self-contained units such as those used in the juvenile studies. In the large prison systems, these small-group processes may become overwhelmed or contaminated by experiences and issues involving the general population of prisoners. The fact, however, that alienation and inmate solidarity in opposition to staff varies significantly among different prisons and prison systems indicates the need to undertake comparative studies to identify the critical variables and subject them to experimental control.

The inmate subcultures and prisonization theories about prison life have been criticized for their neglect of individual differences in the way prisoners cope with the conditions and stresses of life in confinement (Porporino and Zamble, 1984). Measures of coping processes were found to be more highly correlated with the development of depressive and anxiety reactions and disciplinary problems than such factors as type of offense, prior prison experience, or criminal history. Poor coping in prison was also found to be related to maladapted functioning in the community following release from imprisonment (Porporino and Zamble, 1984). The value of greater attention to differences in the reaction of prisoners to prison life as a basis for a more effective classification procedures and changes in the organization of prison conditions has been persuasively presented in the psychological studies reported by Hans Toch (Toch, 1975, 1977). Such psychological studies are best advanced by longitudinal and experimental research that permits the documentation of coping strategies that develop and change as offenders adjust to life in confinement, as contrasted with cross-sectional surveys.

One of the most common criticisms of the use of imprisonment is the charge that prisons are schools for crime. In view of the pervasive public belief in this consequence of prison life, it is surprising that more research has not been done to document the process and the amount of learning that takes place. Most studies show that prisoners undergo a process of induction into prison life during which the first timer learns the rules for survival as promulgated by the staff on the one hand and inmates on the other. Descriptions of prison life make it clear that a great deal of conversational time between inmates is consumed with telling stories of past "scores" and plans for new ones (Irwin, 1970). In the course of such discussions, criminal attitudes, values, and beliefs regarding crime, the criminal justice system, and the world of victims are communicated. This often also involves discussion of the techniques of crime and methods of coping with arrest and its consequences. Because most men in prison have served time previously in prison or jail, much of the learning about crime has already occurred. However, Waller found in his study of discharged and paroled prisoners from the federal penitentiary system of Ontario, Canada, that about half of the men said that

there was something new to be learned about crime in the penitentiaries. . . . [But] when asked whether it was possible to not learn about crime there, 91 per cent of the dischargees and 76 per cent of the parolees, replied in the negative. The principal areas mentioned where knowledge could be "gleaned" were safe breaking, bank robbery, circumventing burglar alarms, picking locks, nullifying electronic gadgets, passing cheques, stealing cars, and techniques of violence. (Waller, 1974, p. 66)

When Waller asked if they had gained something positive from prison, only 6% felt they had, and 12% felt that prison had made them more aggressive and belligerent.

However, the studies of learning experiences in prison have been more focused on the process of prisonization than on the relation of what is learned in prison to postprison conduct. This focus is partly a tribute to the impressive pioneering work of Donald Clemmer (1940) in studying socialization and social organization within a prison in Illinois. He perceived prisonization to be a process of progressive assimilation into the general culture of the prison world, a process likely to make the released offender more criminal on his release. Much later, Wheeler (1961) showed that the progression was not a continuous one, that adherence to staff versus inmate norms of conduct was greater during the first phase of prison life and again greater as the release date became imminent, while during the middle phase, the inmate norms gained greater acceptance. A subsequent study by Garbedian (1963) demonstrated, however, that this U-shaped curve of prisonization held true only for certain offenders less concerned with exploitation relationships and status in the prison world itself.

These studies of socialization and adaptation to prison life have been useful in revealing the variety of ways in which different types of offenders seek to accommodate to the demands of the prison. They have not generally, however, addressed the relation between prisonization and postprison adjustment. In a review of the prisonization studies, Hood and Sparks (1970, p. 234) conclude that the critical question was still unanswered: "Is the reconviction rate of any type of ex-prisoner significantly lower (or higher) than would be expected, given his social background, personality, and criminal career before entering the prison?"

One recent study of prison adjustment and transition to community life found that the "institutionalized" inmates concerned with making out well in prison had greater initial difficulty adjusting to community life in the first few months on parole than the "rebellious" inmates who did their own time (Goodstein, 1976). Glaser's (1964) study of the federal prison system in the United States showed that some offenders profited from prison work experiences in that twice as many successes as failures on parole indicated their use of prison training on their jobs. Waller (1974, p. 88) found in Canada that 20% of his sample still free at 12 months had used prison training in some way, as compared to 29.7% in Glaser's sample at 4 months. But it is clear that much more intensive and carefully designed research is needed to investigate the relationship between prison experiences and subsequent criminality. We do not yet know which types of experiences in prison predispose to crime and which work the other way for different types of offenders.

Because of the recent rapid growth in the population and overcrowding of the prisons, research interest has focused on the effects of being confined under such conditions. The research has employed objective and subjective measures of the impact of crowding obtainable within the prison. For example, it has been found that large open-bay dormitories produce higher clinic utilization and higher blood pressure rates than other alternatives such as single- or double-bunked cells, small dormitories, or large partitioned ones (Gaes, 1985). Furthermore, assault rates are higher in prisons containing dormitories or in prisons where the available space is appreciably less than 60 square feet per inmate (Gaes, 1985). It seems clear that crowding has seriously disruptive effects in heightening tension, converting program or hospital space for housing, and making control and regulation of disputes more difficult.

Here again what is needed is an extension of the inquiry as to the possible effects of living under such conditions on conduct following release. Indicative of the value of such research is the study by Farrington and Nuttall (1980) of the relation between size, overcrowding, and reconviction rates using Home Office statistics gathered in the middle 1960s on 19 prisons in England and Wales. They found that overcrowded prisons were much less effective as measured by the difference between predicted and actual reconviction rates. Furthermore, when the effect of overcrowding was controlled, the correlation between the size of the institution and effectiveness was much reduced. This led to the conclusion that "overcrowding was the factor that was clearly negatively related to effectiveness, not size" (Farrington and Nuttall, 1980, p. 229).

External Relationships

Research studies have consistently shown that most prisoners feel more deeply the deprivation of outside contacts with family and friends than they do the privations imposed by life in prison. This apparently applies to long-term as well as short-term prisoners. For example, Richards (1978) developed a list of 20 problems covering various areas of psychological stress for men in prison. He compared the relative severity rankings of these problems by a small matched sample of long-termers (who had served at least 8 years) and short-termers (who had served less than 18 months). There proved to be a high level of agreement between the two groups on problem severity rankings. But of greater interest was the finding that the five most severe problems concerned relations with the outside world. These were (a) missing somebody, (b) feeling that your life is being wasted, (c) feeling sexually frustrated, (d) missing little "luxuries," and (e) missing social life. In contrast, the five least severe problems were (a) losing your self-confidence, (b) feeling angry with the world, (c) being afraid of dying before you get out, (d) being afraid of going mad, and (e) feeling suicidal (Richards, 1978, p. 167). This study was replicated by Flanagan (1980) in maximum security prisons in New York State with findings closely paralleling those of Richards in England. In addition, Flanagan found that the single most important problem was loss of relationships with family and friends outside the prison. Apparently the passage of time makes this loss harder rather than easier to bear. He noted, "some long-term inmates cauterise these relationships as a means of avoiding the anxiety and despair that accompany the separation. For the majority of prisoners who do not attempt this strategy, however, family ties become a two-edged sword over the years, providing encouragement and support and at the same time making it more difficult to do time" (Flanagan, 1980, p. 155).

The importance of the family is also evident among the concerns that prisoners worry about before release. In his study of discharged and paroled prisoners in Ontario, Waller found that:

Employment was felt to be important: 30 per cent mentioned this as a first concern and 33 per cent as a second. Family was mentioned as the first concern by 64 per cent and as the second by 10 per cent. Managing financially was mentioned by 24 per cent as their first concern, and by 20 per cent as their second. After these came worries about returning to prison, relationships with a common-law wife, and then a place to stay. Employment, of course, applied to everybody, whereas family, particularly in the case of a wife, applied differentially. (1974, p. 68)

Studies by Pauline Morris (1965, 1975) of the families of prisoners in England also document the importance of these relationships both during confinement and following release, especially for those serving their first sentence. About three-fourths of the married first-timers were living with their wives prior to sentence, as compared with half of the married recidivists. Furthermore, most of the married first-timers expected to resume living with their wives and usually did so. The Morris study also explored the deprivations experienced by the families of prisoners and the strains that the separation imposes on the marriage relationship. But most important, it suggested the necessity of doing as much as possible during confinement and immediately after release to strengthen these ties as a support system for preventing a return to crime.

In the United States, the variable of "active family interest" during confinement has been especially useful in the prediction of parole success. In Illinois, both Ohlin (1954) and Glaser (1964) found parole success rates for inmates with evidence of active family interest in the neighborhood of 75%. Glaser (1964) also found a 71% success rate in his study of federal prisoners as compared to 50% among those with no contact with relatives. More recently, in a study of 412 prisoners from a minimum security facility in California, Holt and Miller found that the recidivism rate was lowest among those men who had regular family visits and that only 2% of those with 3 or more regular visitors had to be returned to prison. Having a family to go home to after release was more predictive of parole success than such factors as a waiting job or the amount of release money. In reviewing these and other studies, Homer concluded: "In every comparison category, including those with 3 or more prior commitments, men with more family–social ties have had the fewest parole failures" (1979, p. 48).

In general, however, family relationships during and after confinement have received relatively little research attention, except for small studies and the observations of practitioners engaged in family counseling and therapy. Yet, increasingly, the value of family and friendship networks in self-help programs are gaining recognition for their positive supportive potential (Fishman and Alissi, 1979). Further experimentation with these networks in the reintegration of prisoners into the community should be given much higher priority in research funding.

Effects of Imprisonment After Release

The transition from prison to community life is a difficult experience for many prisoners. The contrast between the regimented life in prison and the obligation to take responsibility for one's own living and work arrangements can be a source of emotional stress. Virtually all follow-up studies report such difficulties. Waller's findings in his study of releases in Canada are quite typical in this respect. He found that nearly 40% of the men experienced such stress, but that it tended to be more characteristic of the parolees than the dischargees.

More parolees experienced anxiety, sleeplessness, and trouble talking to people, felt they looked like an ex-prisoner, had a hard time getting used to things, and experienced disappointment concerning things they had planned to enjoy. More dischargees had a tendency to experience such symptoms as loneliness, hard time remembering, and depression. The finding on loneliness is consistent with the tendency for the dischargees to have fewer friends or family to whom to turn. (Waller, 1974, p. 75)

Waller also found, however, that these symptoms tended to dissipate as the ex-prisoner became more adjusted and settled to life outside. Nevertheless, 13% of the dischargees and 17% of the parolees indicated that at one time or another they felt they would have been better off in prison.

In general, most studies of released prisoners show that this type of stress is less for those with a family to return to and note that their recidivism rates are lower as well. The experience of a labeling or stigmatizing effect is also present initially, though this also tends to wear off or become discounted with time. Waller found that after six months, only a minority felt stigmatized by neighbors, police, or employers, while some felt they even got extra help because of their record.

Perhaps the most difficult problem encountered by the ex-prisoner is obtaining a suitable, steady job. In both the Waller and Glaser studies of federal prisoners in Canada and the United States, the employment problem seemed to be less a matter of stigmatization and more a matter of lack of skills, experience, or a regular work history. A number of projects have been undertaken in an attempt to solve the employment problems of ex-prisoners. In the United States, many of these were supported by the Department of Labor under the provisions of the Manpower Development Act of 1962. The early programs concentrated on job training and vocational counseling, but by the late 1960s had shifted to direct job placement and later on to job creation. The experience with such programs, however, has been generally disappointing. For example, a recent review of the accomplishments of the Targeted Jobs Tax Credit program, passed as part of the Revenue Act of 1978, proved essentially negative (Jacobs, McGahey, and Minion, 1984). The program was designed to assist the hiring and training of hard-core unemployed persons on the job by subsidizing their wages. The evaluation

attributed the negative results in part to a lack of publicity, inefficient administration, and insufficient subsidies; it was also noted that "the program stigmatizes
ex-offenders in an effort to aid them and tax credits like TJTC fail to produce
many new jobs for disadvantaged workers, whether or not they are ex-offenders"
(Jacobs *et al.*, 1984, p. 500).

Another direction of assistance for ex-prisoners has been the provision of transitional financial aid during the early stages of the release period. As mentioned
in Chapter 3, an experiment in Baltimore in the early 1970s tested whether ex-
prisoners would benefit more from financial assistance than from job counseling
and placement following release (Lenihan, 1977). The results showed that the
placement and counseling procedures had no impact on rearrests, but the transfer
payments resulted in an 8% reduction in rearrests compared to those not eligible.
These promising results led to a much larger experiment, designated as the Transitional Aid Research Project (TARP) (Rossi, Berk, and Lenihan, 1980). This
project randomly assigned 4,000 men and women about to be released from prisons in Georgia and Texas to four treatment and two control groups. Treatment
groups 1, 2, and 3 received unemployment benefits lasting 26 weeks for group 1
and 13 weeks for groups 2 and 3. However, the payments to groups 1 and 2 were
reduced dollar for dollar based on their earnings from legitimate employment,
while group 3 was taxed only at 25 cents on the dollar. The fourth treatment group
received only job placement.

The TARP experiment produced interesting findings, which are still being
debated and analyzed. In general the payments resulted in a disincentive to find
employment because they did not compare unfavorably to payments for employment at the low-job-skill level for which many of the offenders could qualify.
Those receiving TARP payments worked, on the average, one-third fewer weeks
than the controls. Generally, also the effect of financial aid on rearrest rates
proved disappointing. However, the number of rearrests was reduced with higher
increments of payment. Such payments appeared to increase the opportunity-
costs of being arrested, giving participants more to lose. Similarly, employment
increased the opportunity-costs of arrests by providing another source of income,
occupying time, and forming a stake in legitimate pursuits. The results showed
that the employed ex-prisoner had fewer arrests than those who were unemployed. What remains to be explored is whether changes in the payment procedures can reduce the disincentive-to-work effect.

The TARP project provides a rich resource of data that continues to be
explored. A study by Liker (1982) has shown that employment can provide major
benefits after release in reducing affective stress, such as feelings of depression,
loneliness, and stigma. By providing a steady income, it can reduce the stress
from economic pressures and provide a source of "self-respect, social contacts,
and structured activity" (Liker, 1982, p. 281). Unemployment was found to feed
on itself in creating stress and reduced interest in finding work, a situation that
undoubtedly encourages illegitimate pursuits for those with a criminal history.
Equating unemployment with a return to crime, however, may oversimplify the
experiences of ex-prisoners. A study of releasees from the correctional facility on

Rikers Island in New York City demonstrated a more complex pattern (Sviridoff and Thompson, 1983). Interviews with 61 adult male misdemeanants showed that low-level employment was often accompanied by crime in some cases, while in others it led to alternating periods of crime and work. Some used the income from crime to supplement employment income, while still others used the employment income to set themselves up in various illegitimate economic activities such as drug sales.

Conclusion

The effects of imprisonment have been studied in many ways. Insights have come from the observations of practitioners involved in the treatment or custodial control of prisoners or counseling with family members. Small pilot studies by researchers using observation and intensive interviews have helped in spotting critical influences on prisoners, developing theoretical propositions for more careful testing, and producing descriptive accounts of life in prison and on parole. Others have undertaken the quantitative analysis of official data or have drawn cross-sectional samples for the acquisition of interview or questionnaire data for analysis of prison and parole problems. It is also apparent from the preceding sections of this chapter that many short-term follow-up studies have been made to evaluate the impact of various prison or parole programs on subsequent conduct. It is also obvious, however, that there is a lack of firm knowledge and many gaps in our understanding of the effects of imprisonment on the achievement of the basic objectives of the criminal justice system and on the prisoners themselves while doing time and after release. Very few of the studies have involved experimental designs or sequential observations over a long enough time to discern accurately the processes taking place and their effects for various subgroups of prisoners. Longer-term studies, including experimental tests, would provide a firmer ground for the development of more effective policies. It is to such issues we turn in the remaining chapter.

8
What Kinds of Longitudinal–Experimental Studies Are Needed?

General Aims

In this report, we have highlighted some of the key issues in the explanation, prevention, and treatment of crime. We are especially concerned with violent crimes, predatory crimes such as robbery, and property offenses such as burglary. Some of the key issues in explanation are: Why does crime increase with age to peak in the teenage years? Why do people stop offending after age 20? How far are the most antisocial people at one age also the most antisocial at another? Why are parental family-management practices the best predictors of delinquency? Why do people start or stop committing crimes? What is the influence of peers on offending? How is school failure linked to offending? What is the effect on offending of events such as leaving school, getting married, and becoming unemployed? Why do criminal parents and low-income families produce delinquent children? What are the effects of official labeling on crime (Chapter 5)?

Some of the key issues in prevention and treatment are: Can delinquency be prevented by parent training or by a preschool intellectual enrichment program (Chapter 4)? Can delinquency be prevented by exposure to a prosocial peer group (Chapter 3)? How far can "chronic" offenders be predicted? What are the effects of diverting offenders from the court (Chapter 5)? What are the effects on offending of juvenile as opposed to adult court processing (Chapter 6)? What are the effects on adult court decision making of providing juvenile records? What are the effects of different sentences on offenders? What interactions are there between the effectiveness of correctional treatments and types of offenders (Chapter 3)? What are the effects of imprisonment on prisoners (Chapter 7)? Can the recidivism rate of released prisoners be reduced by providing welfare benefits or special assistance with employment?

We believe that the best method of advancing knowledge about these (and other) key issues is by means of longitudinal–experimental surveys. As explained earlier, in these kinds of studies, people are followed up over a period, and the effects on them of experimental interventions at different times are investigated. In this chapter, we will set out general principles for desirable longitudinal–experimental surveys. The examples we have chosen are meant to be illustrative rather than prescriptive. The kinds of projects proposed here have never before been attempted in the field of criminology.

Longitudinal–experimental surveys on crime have two distinct aims. The first is to establish the course of development of criminal careers—in particular, the prevalence and incidence of different crimes at different ages, leading to specification of the onset, duration, and termination of offending. The second is to establish the effects of specific events on the course of development of criminal careers in order to test hypotheses about what causes criminal behavior and about what can prevent it before and reduce it after it occurs. This aim involves studying the impact of interventions on specific features of criminal careers in the context of long-term information about development.

The arguments in favor of longitudinal–experimental surveys have been stated earlier in this report and will not be repeated here. Because these surveys have two different elements and two different aims, they can be used for both generating and testing hypotheses about crime. However, as indicated in Chapter 2, other methods often can and should be used to generate hypotheses that are not specifically concerned with the time course of criminal careers.

In devising longitudinal–experimental surveys, there are many choices that have to be made. Time and resources are always limited. The choices we make inevitably reflect our assessment of the best answers to questions such as the following: Should one cohort or several be followed up and for how long? What kinds of people should be studied? Where should the project be carried out? How should the data be collected? What factors should be measured at different ages? What kinds of experimental manipulations should be tested? These kinds of questions will be discussed in detail in the sections "Design Choices," "Cohorts to Be Followed," and "Possible Interventions," and we will make some specific suggestions about how they might be answered.

In the section "Subsidiary Issues," we will discuss the need for preparatory research, supplementary smaller-scale studies, the need for replication, the use of quasi-experimental analyses, and research on larger units than individuals (such as areas, schools, and penal institutions). The value of quasi-experimental analyses and of research on larger units has been discussed in Chapters 2 and 3.

Design Choices

One or Several Cohorts?

Our major interest is in studying the development of criminal careers from birth to the mid-twenties. This period covers the onset of offending, the peak age for prevalence, the peak period of commission of the kinds of offenses in which we are interested (roughly ages 14 to 21), and the beginning of the decline in prevalence with age. One obvious way of investigating this would be to follow up one cohort from birth to age 24 (for example). However, there are many problems with this single cohort approach.

First of all, the research would take a generation to complete. It might be difficult to ensure continuity in directing the research because the principal investigators would age at the same rate as the subjects. Also, it would undoubtedly be difficult to secure a funding commitment for such a long-term project. Obviously, the key results might be delayed too long for the liking of funding agencies (especially those controlled by short-lived political appointees) who want to see results within a few years. Also, in a very-long-term project, problems may be caused by changes in theories, methods, and policy concerns. Key issues at the start of a long-term survey might be considered unimportant by the end, and the latest methods at the start might be regarded as outdated by the end. In addition, attrition and mobility cause increasing difficulty as the length of a survey is extended.

Another major problem with the traditional long-term survey is the confusion of aging, period, and cohort effects. The British National Survey, for example, followed up a sample of children born in March 1946 (Wadsworth, 1979). To what extent were changes seen in these children between age 10 in 1956 and age 21 in 1967 a reflection of *aging* from 10 to 21? To what extent were they a feature of this particular *cohort*, who were at the peak of the postwar baby boom, and therefore competing for resources to a much greater degree than those born in 1954, for example? To what extent were they a reflection of changes during the *period* 1956–1967? Some cohorts are clearly subject to unique and perhaps unpredictable influences. For example, the cohort of Polk *et al.* (1981) were those who went to fight in the Vietnam War. On the one hand, it is interesting to study the effects of unique historical events; on the other hand, this limits the extent to which the results can be generalized.

At the other extreme, the development of criminal careers from birth to age 24 could be studied by following up 24 cohorts for one year, beginning with every age from birth to age 23. However, this method also has many disadvantages. Assuming that it is desirable to establish developmental trends before and after an experimental intervention, a one-year total period is too short. Unrealistically frequent interviews would be required, and there may be very little developmental change over such a short period. In any case, some experimental interventions do not occur at one point in time but may extend over several months or even a year (e.g., a preschool intellectual enrichment program). A one-year period is too short to investigate continuity and change over time, given the likely speed of developmental change. Also, it is too short to study developmental sequences of events, where a change in one factor can be shown (quasi-experimentally) to be followed by a change in another.

It might be thought that conclusions could be drawn about long-term predictability or continuity by linking up cohorts. For example, in studying the time course of criminal careers, we might be interested in relating the number of offenses committed at age 15 to the number committed at age 16, age 17, age 18, age 19, and so on up to age 24. Rather than following up one cohort from age 15 to age 24, we could follow up nine cohorts from age 15 to age 16, age 16 to age 17, age 17 to age 18, and so on. However, a major problem with the multiple cohort approach is statistical fluctuation or sampling variation. Given the likely number who could be interviewed at each age, confidence intervals for measures would be quite wide. The single cohort approach is better because each person acts as his or her own control, thus reducing the variability of measures.

These considerations indicate that the best compromise is to follow up a few cohorts for a few years. As an example, we will propose that four cohorts each be followed up for six years: from birth to age 6, from 6 to 12, from 12 to 18, and from 18 to 24. These age ranges are chosen for illustrative purposes, but they will be justified in the section "Cohorts to Be Followed," where the cohorts are discussed in more detail. These six-year periods are sufficiently short for the project to be practically feasible but sufficiently long to study continuity and developmental change and to build up a complete picture of development from birth to age 24. If resources permitted, some of the original cohorts could be followed up after the end of the six-year period, and some new cohorts could be followed up between the same ages in order to disentangle aging and period effects.

The choice of these six-year follow-up periods is to some extent arbitrary. However, this design is, in our view, a reasonable compromise between the 24-year follow-up of one cohort and the one-year follow-up of 24 cohorts (which is similar to a cross-sectional survey). The longitudinal survey is needed to investigate continuity and developmental changes over time, developmental sequences in which one event precedes another, and the general issue of prediction. It is needed, for example, to study the extent of switching from one type of crime to another and the extent to which the onset or persistence of offending can be predicted.

The longitudinal survey is especially needed to investigate the effects of specific events, such as experimental manipulations, on the time course of criminal careers. It is desirable to establish trends over time before the manipulation is introduced, as pointed out in the discussion of Murray and Cox (1979) in Chapter 3. In view of the likely speed of developmental change between birth and age 24, a six-year follow-up period with experimental manipulations somewhere in the middle seems a reasonable compromise. Even with this length of follow-up, there may be a period of 10 years from the start of a project to the publication of the full results, allowing time for preparatory and pilot work before the data collection begins and time for analysis and writing up after the data collection ends. Of course, it is likely that some useful results could be published long before the end of the project, from the first year or two of data collection, for example.

An advantage of linking together a number of short-term longitudinal–experimental surveys is that it might be possible to draw conclusions about long-term effects of interventions. This assumes that the longitudinal samples are large enough to overcome the problem of statistical fluctuation mentioned earlier. For example, imagine that in the survey from birth to age 6, a preschool intellectual enrichment program at ages 3 to 4 produced an improvement in school behavior at age 6. The survey from 6 to 12 may well show how school behavior at 6 predicts school behavior at 12, while the survey from 12 to 18 may show how school behavior at 12 predicts delinquency by 18, and the survey from 18 to 24 may show how delinquency by 18 predicts adult offending by 24. Would it not be reasonable to conclude from this chain of evidence that a preschool intellectual enrichment program has a long-term crime reducing effect? This could of course be verified by longer-term follow-ups of the original birth cohort, once the basic result had been obtained.

Target Population

In deciding what kinds of people to study, the major choice is between a sample from the general population, a "high-risk" sample, and a sample of offenders.

The main advantage of following up a general population sample is that the results can be widely generalized. This is the best method of identifying the proportion of the population who commit different kinds of crimes, for example. Furthermore, since all segments of the population are studied, knowledge is gained about all the various subgroups who are substantially represented in the population—males and females, whites, blacks, and hispanics, urban, suburban, and rural subjects. The main disadvantage of the general-population sample is that the number of frequent and serious offenders is likely to be very small. Therefore, this sample provides only limited information about those persons who are the greatest threat to society and who are our main concern. Also, the number of persons in a random sample from minority groups in the population will be small.

One way of providing more information about the most frequent and serious offenders is to study a sample drawn from those subgroups of the general population who are most at risk of becoming such offenders. A sample of black urban males could be followed up, for example. Alternatively, infrequent groups in the population could be oversampled, such as blacks, hispanics, or children in one-parent families. The increased yield of frequent, serious offenders would be purchased at the cost of a decreased ability to generalize to the whole population, but the ability to generalize to the population of frequent, serious offenders would be improved. Conclusions drawn from a sample of black urban males about the onset, duration, and termination of criminal careers, or about the effects of events on the course of development of such careers, might not apply to other subgroups in the population, of course.

Another method of obtaining reliable information about frequent and serious offenders would be to limit the sample to only detected offenders. For example, a sample of persons arrested for the first time, convicted for the first time, or imprisoned for the first time could be followed up. However, the increased knowledge about frequent, serious offenders would again be purchased at the cost of a decreased ability to generalize to the whole population. In particular, nothing would be known about the extent of offending by nonarrested offenders. This information is important, for example, in establishing the effect on overall crime rates of a policy of incapacitation of serious offenders.

One way of identifying a high-risk nonarrested group would be to choose young people with high self-reported offending scores who had not been apprehended. This would require a two-stage process of selection of the sample, which is often a useful strategy. In the first stage, a short and inexpensive screening question-naire could be given to a large sample of potential subjects in the general popula-tion; the results obtained could then be used in selecting those who would be studied more intensively (and expensively) in the second stage. This kind of suc-cessive screening was recommended by Loeber, Dishion, and Patterson (1984). Carefully used, it could maximize the yield of frequent serious offenders while still making it possible to generalize to the whole population.

This discussion illustrates a general point. Every decision about research design has advantages and disadvantages. Because resources are always limited, it is never possible to carry out the perfect research project. The solution adopted here is to recommend several linked projects carried out in the same area. If a general-population cohort is followed up, together with a "high-risk" cohort, together with an arrest cohort, and together with a prison cohort coming from the same area, it should be possible to link all the data to build up a complete picture both of the general population and of the most frequent and serious offenders within it. This kind of extensive linking of data from different projects in the same area has not been attempted before in the field of criminology.

Location of Research

In regard to location, the major choice is between local, national, and interna-tional projects.

The major advantages of a local project are practical. It is much easier to carry out a study in one Standard Metropolitan Statistical Area (SMSA) than a national study. It is very difficult to establish, maintain, and control the quality of a nationwide system of interviewers, for example, although this was achieved in the national study by Elliott et al. (1983). More important, it would be almost impossible to investigate the effects of experimental manipulations in a national study because of the cost and difficulty of setting up experiments throughout the United States.

The most extensive existing criminological experiment is probably the TARP study of Rossi et al. (1980). As described in Chapter 3, this provided unemploy-ment benefit payments to ex-prisoners. The experiment cost $3,400,000, and involved nearly 4,000 prisoners in two states (Georgia and Texas). Other states were considered but eliminated either because they were unwilling to carry out the random assignment or because they had incomplete or noncomputerized criminal justice information systems. This study gives some idea of what might be feasible as a criminological experiment.

If a project was based in one SMSA, the subjects could be selected by cluster sampling. In other words, only a limited number of areas within the city would be selected as project areas, although the aim would be to generalize to the whole city. It would be possible to build into this design some stratified sampling of high-risk or minority areas in order to increase the amount of information gained about the most frequent and serious offenders.

An advantage of a local project is that the context of the research can be studied in detail. Extensive information can be collected about the characteristics of local areas, community resources, local schools, police and court practices, and institutional provision. Key persons in the areas can be interviewed—police chiefs and other criminal justice personnel, teachers, social agency representatives, and community leaders. The behavior of the subjects of any study is likely to be better understood if it can be placed in its social context, especially when this social context varies a great deal from one area to another—as in the United States. To take an obvious example, the likelihood of committing a crime depends to some extent on the pattern of opportunities for crime. This pattern could be established in a local study but not in a national one. In fact, it would be virtually impossible to collect detailed contextual information in a national study [see also the section "Supplementary Studies"].

The major disadvantage of a local study in comparison with a national one is the limited ability to generalize. A critic could always argue that results obtained in Philadelphia, for example, would not apply in Los Angeles or New York City. However, a counterargument would be that national data are not necessarily applicable to any particular area. The best solution is probably to begin in one SMSA with the intention of replicating key results subsequently in others.

The cross-sectional survey by Tittle (1980a) is an example of a project based on a small number of areas. He was interested in studying deterrence by relating self-reports of offending to perceptions about the probability of being caught and punished, and he interviewed about 2,000 randomly selected adults in three states. Tittle divided all the states into three groups and selected New Jersey as representative of the urban–industrial group, Oregon of the moderately urban–industrial group, and Iowa of the rural–nonindustrial group. In this way, although he only studied three states, he had some reflection of the diversity across the whole country.

From the viewpoint of mounting longitudinal–experimental studies, a state would be too large a unit because of the diversity and distance within it. This is one of the reasons why an SMSA is proposed. Another reason is that the crime problem is more acute in the large cities. In the context of national crime policy, it is more important to study the causes, prevention, and treatment of crimes in the large cities. Research is likely to be more difficult and indeed dangerous in these cities, but the greater yield of frequent and serious offenders justifies the risk.

The choice of SMSAs to study depends on a number of factors, and the three largest SMSAs (New York, Chicago, and Los Angeles) are not necessarily the best choices. One of the most important considerations is the willingness of criminal justice and other agencies to cooperate in experimentation. Another is the adequacy and accessibility of existing records, inasmuch as the first stage in any study is likely to involve the extraction of data from records (especially criminal justice records). Another important consideration is the existence of a competent research team in the area with experience in longitudinal or experimental research. There would be advantages in trying to compare newly collected data with longitudinal information about criminal histories in past years, where this is available, to study changes over relatively long time periods.

Another important problem is mobility. If the population of an SMSA is highly mobile, the advantages of a local study will have been lost within a few years because of the dispersal of the sample. Although it is possible to follow up by means of interviews those who move, it is more difficult to include them in any experiment. Therefore, if a sample is highly mobile, there is the danger that the experimental manipulations conducted in the city itself will be carried out on possibly unrepresentative subsamples. This may limit the generalizability or external validity of the results, but it does not threaten their internal validity. Providing that persons are randomly assigned to experimental and control groups, those in the experimental group will be just as likely to move before the experimental manipulation as those in the control group, so the two groups should still be comparable at the time of the experimental manipulation. However, it is desirable to choose an SMSA with low mobility or at least to avoid cities such as Miami with a high rate of in-and-out migration. Another way of trying to cope with mobility would be to make experimental manipulations as portable as possible, but this may not be easy.

Initially, projects should be limited to the United States. However, there would be advantages later in planning for some international comparisons. From the viewpoint of assessing sociocultural influences, it is important to establish how far key results can be replicated in different cultures. It is interesting that many of the results obtained by Robins (1979) in the United States have been replicated by Farrington and West (1981) in England, and an illuminating comparison of official criminal history records in Philadelphia and Copenhagen has been completed by Van Dusen and Mednick (1983).

It would be best if international comparisons were restricted to metropolitan areas. Similar longitudinal–experimental studies could be mounted in cities outside the United States that fulfill some of the criteria outlined above. For example, there are research teams with the necessary expertise located in London, Copenhagen, and Stockholm, which would all be reasonable possibilities for comparison with large American cities.

Demographic Characteristics of Subjects

A great deal of criminological research and theory in the past has been concerned primarily with lower-class, young urban males. It is only in recent years that females have been studied more extensively, and it is still true that there is little research on crimes by middle- or upper-class people, older people, or those living in rural areas. The concentration on lower-class, young urban males reflects the belief that they are responsible for the most frequent and serious offending. Therefore, as usual, there is a tradeoff between obtaining information that is applicable to the whole population and obtaining data on the most frequent and serious offenders.

It will be clear from the section "Location of Research" that we are proposing longitudinal–experimental studies based initially in one SMSA; to that extent, the problem of crime in rural areas will not be addressed. Equally, in the section "Cohorts to Be Followed" we will propose projects designed to illuminate the development of offending from birth up to the twenties, and therefore it follows that crime by middle-aged and older people will not be studied.

It is never possible to study everything in any one project or even in a series of linked projects such as proposed here. Choices have to be made, and they can limit the ability to generalize. There are two major justifications for concentrating on crimes by young people in urban areas. One is that, since most is known about these kinds of crimes, it is easiest to put forward plausible hypotheses about events that may affect the course of development of these people's careers. Experiments are essentially designed to test hypotheses. Because there is less research on older people and rural areas, there would be less empirical justification for hypotheses about influences on rural or adult criminal careers. The second reason has already been stated in this section—namely, the belief that young people in urban areas commit the most frequent and serious offenses.

Within the limitation of urban young people, it would be desirable to study males and females and the major ethnic groups present in the cities (normally whites, blacks, and hispanics). It is important to establish how features of criminal careers vary over these groups and whether interventions have different effects with different sexes or ethnic groups. Limited resources may force an initial concentration on males only, because males are much more likely to become frequent and serious offenders. However, an alternative strategy would be to study both males and females, but only those who pass through an initial screening filter for potential high-rate offenders.

Although the projects proposed here are concerned with young people, it would be quite feasible to extend them to study older people, if resources were available. This could be achieved either by following up existing samples to later ages or by drawing new samples of older people from the same areas. Equally, it would be possible in principle to replicate the projects in rural areas.

Data Collection Decisions

One of the first data collection decisions that has to be made concerns the size of the sample. Again, there is a tradeoff. Large samples of many thousands have advantages in estimating population values with small confidence intervals. For example, if the prevalence of arrests in a sample of 100 people was 25%, there would be a 95% probability that the true population prevalence was within 8.5% of this figure (i.e., between 16.5 and 33.5%)—rather a wide confidence interval. If the prevalence in a sample of 1,000 was 25%, the 95% confidence interval for the population prevalence would be $25 \pm 2.7\%$—a much narrower confidence interval. If the prevalence in a sample of 10,000 was 25%, the 95% confidence interval for the population prevalence would be $25 \pm 0.8\%$—narrower still.

The obvious disadvantage of large samples of many thousands is that the cost of repeated face-to-face interviews becomes considerable. This is why the existing longitudinal studies of many thousands have never attempted these kinds of interviews but have limited themselves to the extraction of information from records (e.g., Wolfgang *et al.*, 1972) or have taken advantage of data collected by persons who would be seeing the subjects anyway (e.g., school teachers and health visitors in the study of Wadsworth,1979). The largest sample that has been interviewed repeatedly in a long-term criminological study is the 1,700 of Elliott *et al.* (1983), but repeated interviews are rare with samples of more than 1,000.

We advocate a sample size of about 1,000 for each cohort study, as the best compromise between the largest sample that could be interviewed repeatedly (given foreseeable resources) and the smallest that would have anything approaching acceptable confidence intervals for population values. Of course, in order to secure 1,000 interviews, the initial target sample would have to be larger. For example, in the victimization survey by Farrington and Dowds (1985), an issued sample of 1,330 randomly chosen households in each of three English counties led to an average of just over 1,000 interviews with adults in each county. (The aim was to interview one randomly chosen adult in each household.) In view of the plan for repeated interviews, and the likelihood of attrition, the initial target sample for each cohort might have to be 1,500.

Assuming that the cohorts are to be drawn from households, many more than 1,500 households would have to be screened to locate subjects of the desired ages. Other sampling frames, such as schools, are possible. However, the main advantage of deriving all cohorts from households is that they can be linked together more easily. Another advantage is economy in drawing samples because the same household can be screened at the same time for eligible persons in different cohorts.

The next data collection decisions concern the types of information to be collected and the rate of contact. We have advocated that it is desirable to collect data from a variety of sources to distinguish results that reflect the theoretical construct of interest from those that reflect biases specific to one method. We have also advocated that repeated face-to-face interviews are desirable, preferably at intervals of not more than one year, although this would depend on the speed of developmental change. In addition to regular interviewing, it would be desirable to arrange for data collection to be triggered by special events (such as arrest, marriage, or a general social change such as the closure of a factory that affected the whole community).

In addition to interviewing, data should be collected from available records and from key informants such as parents, teachers, peers, employers, and criminal justice personnel. Attempts should be made to collect information by direct observation, possibly in supplementary smaller-scale studies [see the section "Supplementary Studies"]. Data could be collected much more frequently in such studies. For example, Patterson (1980a) investigated parent–child interactions by direct observation and also evaluated his treatment methods using daily telephone calls to get parental reports of the child's stealing in the previous 24 hours. He was able to show that his behavioral treatment led to a significant decrease in reported stealing over a five-week period, which then persisted during a six-month follow-up.

Telephone interviews and mail questionnaires could be used as an inexpensive way of collecting data between expensive face-to-face interviews. Another way of reducing the cost would be to interview subsamples of the main sample at different ages, again possibly in between attempts to contact the whole sample. However, there are obvious disadvantages in not having complete data on the whole sample. The lack of complete data is not so serious in regard to the estimation of quantities such as the prevalence rate at different ages, but it does have serious effects on attempts to plot or predict the course of development of criminal careers, on studies of continuity or discontinuity, and on attempts to establish the effects of specific events on this course of development.

The variables that might be measured will differ at different ages and in different cohorts. They will be discussed in more detail in the section "Cohorts to Be Followed." However, considerable effort should be made in all studies to measure offending through records, self-reports, and reports from key informants. In some cases, it may be possible to measure offending by direct observation. As an example of this, Buckle and Farrington (1984) observed persons shoplifting in a department store. Direct observation of offending may be most feasible with persons in penal institutions. Graham (1981) measured the breaking of cell windows by direct observation and showed that it could be reduced by increasing the likelihood of detection and punishment.

It is also desirable to measure the circumstances in which offenses occur and, in particular, whether offenses are committed in groups or alone. As pointed out in Chapter 2, this affects estimates of how many different crimes have been committed. It is also important to measure noncriminal deviant behavior that is often associated with offending, such as truancy, lying, destructiveness, bullying, running away, fighting, and rebellious behavior (for children) and excessive drinking, drug taking, heavy gambling, dangerous driving, and sexual promiscuity (for adults). As indicated in Chapter 2, people tend to be versatile not only in the variety of offenses they commit but also in the commission of other kinds of deviant acts. It would be useful to know about noncriminal acts that lead to criminal acts in developmental sequences from the point of view of possibly intervening early in the sequence.

Planning for Continued Contact

Attrition has always been a major problem in longitudinal surveys. It is made worse in criminological surveys by the fact that the most uncooperative and elusive subjects tend also to be the most delinquent and criminal and, hence, the most interesting. Maintaining contact over six years is a less daunting prospect than maintaining contact over 24 years; even so, it is essential that researchers plan from the beginning how to maintain contact with the maximum possible number of people in the sample, especially with the highest-risk subjects. Ideally, the cooperation of whole communities should be enlisted. One possible strategy is to explain in great detail to every subject at the start about every aspect of the survey and to accept as subjects only those who promise that they will participate throughout. However, this can lead to a serious loss of subjects, threatening the representativeness of the final sample. For example, when Loeber and Dishion (1984) explained their extensive data collection procedures to 1,000 families in Oregon, only 300 were willing to participate.

The two major causes of losing subjects are failure to locate them and their own uncooperativeness after being located. There are various ways of minimizing both of these problems. In regard to minimizing difficulties in locating people, one strategy has already been discussed. The area of the research should be chosen carefully, and areas with low mobility and cooperative agencies are best. It is also desirable to collect as much identifying information about each person at the start of the study as possible, including not only the full name, address, and date of birth of the subject but also the names and addresses of parents, other relatives, friends, and employers. Subjects can be located from telephone directories (the cheapest and easiest method, provided the approximate area is known), electoral registers, records (e.g., criminal, motor vehicle, medical), agencies (e.g., the post office, institutions, schools, professional tracing firms), or from friends, relatives, occupants of previous addresses, or neighbors.

In order to maintain cooperation, it is desirable to warn the subjects at the start that continued cooperation is wanted and to reinforce participation throughout. Ideally, the subjects should be made to feel part of an important enterprise, interested in the project, and given regular feedback about the results. Unfortunately, the most uncooperative and criminal persons may not be receptive to these kinds of arguments but might be persuaded by payments, gifts, or other benefits. Even a regular birthday card to subjects can help! In general, regular contact helps both in locating subjects and in maintaining cooperation.

Cohorts to Be Followed

General Design

As already indicated in the section "One or Several Cohorts?," the illustrative design involves following several cohorts, drawn from the same area, over a six-year period: from birth, from age 6, from age 12, and from age 18. In addition to these population cohorts, it is suggested that a cohort of arrested persons be followed from age 15 to age 21, assuming that the minimum age for adult court in the area is 18; and that a cohort of persons drawn from the area, aged 18 to 24, and beginning their first prison sentences, should also be followed for six years. Each cohort could consist of about 1,000 persons interviewed. Similarly, each cohort could consist ideally of males and females and the main ethnic groups in the area (probably whites, blacks, and hispanics). However, some cohorts might have to consist of males only (e.g., the prison cohort, in view of the small number of females in American prisons).

As explained in the section "Design Choices," the emphasis is on linking results from different cohorts to build up a complete picture of the development of criminal careers from birth to young adulthood. The arrested and prison cohorts will provide more detailed information about the frequent and serious offenders, but it should still be possible to link them to the other cohorts. The arrested and prison cohorts should in general be found to be at the extremes of the normal population cohorts.

As explained earlier, there are two aims in following up each cohort. The first is to establish features of criminal careers such as prevalence and incidence rates at different ages, and the relation between earlier and later events, in a control group who are not subject to any manipulations. The second is to establish the effects of experimental manipulations, which will be proposed in the section "Possible Interventions," on the course of development of these careers. The following sections give a brief indication of the types of factors that might be measured in the various projects.

The Birth Cohort

It is desirable to follow up a cohort from birth in order to investigate whether events that occur in the first few years of life have important effects on later antisocial and criminal behavior. In the early years, data could be collected by interviewing parents and by home observations. When the children are aged 5 to 6, they can be interviewed or tested in kindergarten or in elementary school, and ratings can then be obtained from their teachers. The main factors to be measured are behavior, temperament, attitudes, and abilities, with special reference to conduct disorders such as stealing, aggression, lying, fighting, restlessness, and destructiveness. Also, nervous habits should be measured, including fears and sleep disturbances, and medical factors such as low birth weight and perinatal problems. In addition, parental characteristics, child-rearing behavior (discipline and supervision), and attitudes should be measured as well as parental agreement and the incidence of child abuse and family violence.

The School-Entry Cohort

A cohort could be followed up from age 6 to age 12 to investigate the extent to which events during the elementary school years affect later antisocial, delinquent, and criminal behavior. In addition, efforts should be made to assess the age of onset of different types of offending and antisocial behaviors during this period. Many researchers have demonstrated that an early age of onset of official processing for offending (under age 12) tends to predict later serious and persistent criminal behavior (e.g., Loeber, 1982), but surprisingly little detailed information has been published about prevalence and incidence rates during these years or about the linkage between offending and other kinds of problem behavior.

The major factors to be measured are child behavior (especially antisocial and offending behavior), attitudes, intelligence, and attainment, and parental characteristics, child-rearing behavior, and attitudes as detailed above. Information can be collected from the children themselves, from their parents, from their teachers, and from their peers.

The Adolescent Cohort

It is proposed that a cohort of children also be followed from age 12 to age 18. This period of life has always been recognized as crucial for the development of delinquency and crime, encompassing as it does the peak age of offending (at least in terms of prevalence). It is believed that this period is notable for a gradual disengagement from the family of origin and a corresponding increase in peer influence. More criminological research has studied this age period than any other, and more theories have been proposed about it than about any other. Clearly, any longitudinal–experimental study must include it.

Information should be collected about all aspects of criminal careers including prevalence, incidence, and age of onset for different kinds of offenses. Regular data collection is especially important with this age range because it is believed to be a period of rapid developmental change in offending and in other aspects of life. Information should also be sought about other kinds of deviant activities (such as drinking, smoking, drug use, reckless driving, truancy, running away, fighting, gambling, and sexual promiscuity), about relationships with the family, peer groups, and members of the opposite sex, about school attainments, and (during the later part of the period) about early employment history. Data can be collected from the juveniles themselves, from their parents, from their teachers, and from their peers.

Because most existing criminological theories are primarily concerned with this age range, special attempts should be made in this study to collect data that would permit the testing of major theories. For example, in order to study the theory of Elliott et al. (1985), which to a large extent integrates earlier sociological explanations, attachments to family, school, peers, and work should be measured as well as aspirations for status and material rewards. In order to test the more psychological theory proposed by Wilson and Herrnstein (1985), decision making in criminal opportunities should be investigated, with special reference to the perceived benefits (such as material gain and peer approval), the perceived costs (such as feelings of guilt arising from the conscience and legal punishments), and the extent to which people are influenced by immediate as opposed to future consequences. The measurement of the constructs included in these two recent theories would probably make it possible to test most others. For example, in studying Glaser's (1978) differential-anticipation theory, it would be necessary to measure social bonds as in the Elliott et al. (1985) theory and the costs and benefits of offending as in the Wilson and Hernstein (1985) theory.

The Young Adult Cohort

In most jurisdictions, the age of 18 marks the transition from juvenile to adult legal status. Between 18 and 24, the prevalence of offending declines sharply. This decline is believed to reflect the declining influence of the peer group during these years and the corresponding increase in the influence of marriage or cohabitation, a new family, and conventional institutions such as employment. It is important to establish the causes of the decline in offending in some detail. Little is known about factors that influence the termination of criminal careers.

Information should be collected about the criminal and deviant behavior of the subjects, about their employment history, about their involvement with the peer group, and about their history of relationships with the opposite sex. Data should also be collected about their spouses and cohabitees, about family violence and the quality of their marriages, and (when they become parents) about their own child-rearing behavior and child abuse. Ideally, the subjects and their spouses or cohabitees should be interviewed. It is likely that problems of tracing subjects will be especially acute in this study because the period from 18 to 24 is marked by great mobility. Special efforts may have to be made to gain cooperation and maintain involvement.

The Arrested Cohort

It is proposed that a cohort of arrested (or possibly convicted) persons aged 15 should be followed up to age 21. This will cover the period before and after the transition from juvenile to adult court, assuming that this occurs at age 18. The advantage of following up arrested persons is that more information will be gained about serious and frequent offending during and immediately following the peak age. The key questions to be investigated concern the prediction of high-rate offenders out of all offenders, the effects of different methods of dealing with detected offenders, the stigmatizing effects of official processing (Chapter 5), and the effects of being dealt with by the juvenile as opposed to the adult criminal justice system (Chapter 6). An advantage of beginning at 15 is that it will be possible to obtain juvenile arrest records since these may be destroyed at 18.

It may be desirable to narrow down this cohort to persons arrested for certain types of offenses. From the viewpoint of public policy, it would be most interesting to study violent juvenile offenders. There would be advantages in tracking 15-year-olds who were experiencing their first arrest (so that their complete arrest history could be followed), but this would have the disadvantage of excluding the more serious juvenile offenders who had been arrested at earlier ages. If the focus of interest was the impact of the first arrest, another strategy would be to follow a sample of nonarrested 15-year-olds with a high risk of arrest (for example, with high self-reported offending scores). If a cohort was defined at the time of arrest (e.g., a consecutive sample of arrestees), this might allow a better study of group offending than in a household cohort because the arrest cohort could include all members of offending groups.

The variables to be measured would in general be those outlined above in the teenage and young adult cohorts, but special efforts would be made to inquire about the subjects' experiences, knowledge, attitudes, and perceptions about different aspects of the juvenile and criminal justice systems. Efforts would also be made to link up and compare results obtained in this project with those obtained in the teenage and young adult population cohorts.

The Prison Cohort

A cohort of persons (probably all male), drawn from the area, aged 18 to 24, and beginning their first prison sentences, should also be followed up for six years. The major justification for this study is that the effects of imprisonment and of postprison measures have not been established in well-designed, methodologically adequate studies such as those proposed here (see Chapter 7). Imprisonment, of course, is perhaps the costliest and most important criminal sanction and also in many cases the ultimate deterrent.

It may be necessary to narrow down the definition of the cohort in light of the policy issues that are perceived as most salient. If the interest is in the relation between preprison, prison, and postprison behavior, it would be desirable to restrict the sample to those serving less than a certain length of time, to ensure that they would have both a period in prison and a period after release in the community within the follow-up period. If the interest is in the adjustment after release of long-term prisoners, it may be better to define the sample as a released cohort rather than an entering cohort. If the interest is in the impact of the first prison sentence, this would require the exclusion of those who had been in prison before (and possibly also those who had been in jails or juvenile institutions). One solution to these conflicting demands would be to have different subsamples within the prison cohort. For example, half could be entering prisoners at the start of the study and the other half could be prisoners nearing release.

The factors to be measured would fall into two classes—namely, those measured in prison and those measured after release. On reception into prison, questions should be asked about preprison behavior and attitudes. The major variables measured in prison would be the person's behavior (especially in relation to prison offenses), attitudes (especially to offending and the law), and capabilities (assuming that it is important to investigate the possibility of deterioration as well as the acquisition of new skills in prison). In addition, the person's relationships with other prisoners, with guards, and with family and friends outside should be measured as well as aspects of the prison environment such as the degree of crowding and living conditions. After release, the person's offending and deviant behavior should be studied together with indexes of social adjustment such as employment and marriage or cohabitation history.

Data can be collected from the prisoners themselves, from guards, from employers, and from wives or cohabitees. A major aim would be to link up and compare results obtained in this cohort with those obtained in the young adult population.

Possible Interventions

General Design

The aim should be to assign persons in a cohort at random either to experience one intervention at some stage or to be controls who do not experience any intervention. The advantage of restricting the number of interventions to one for each experimental subject is that it avoids the problem of possible interactions between interventions or the fact that a person's course of development may have already been changed by the first intervention. The aim would be to establish the effect of one intervention on the normal course of development of criminal careers. The controls would be followed up to establish the natural history of development in the absence of the experimental intervention.

The relative proportion of control and experimental subjects depends to some extent on the number of different interventions and on the perceived relative importance of information about criminal careers as opposed to information about effects of interventions. The more the concern about natural history, the higher should be the proportion of control subjects. One possibility is that half of each sample should be controls, that a quarter should experience one intervention, and that the remaining quarter should experience a second intervention.

There are various tradeoffs to be considered in regard to the interventions. For example, the more elements that there are in an intervention, the better is the chance of having an effect on the criminal career, but the greater is the problem of establishing precisely which elements were effective and the greater is the difficulty of replicating any observed effect. In view of the fact that, historically, the problem has been to demonstrate any effect at all, we propose that researchers should not be too worried about the heterogeneity of interventions. If an intervention has a significant effect, it is always possible to carry out subsequent research to establish the separate (or even interactive) effects of the different elements of it.

Another tradeoff is between trying to provide exactly the same intervention for each experimental subject and allowing the strength or intensity of the intervention to vary so that it is subsequently possible (given an overall significant effect) to establish the relation between intensity and effectiveness. In practice, it is difficult to provide interventions that are exactly the same for each person, just as it is difficult not to provide heterogeneous interventions, so there is some force in the argument that variations in intensity should be planned rather than unplanned. Similarly, the ages at which interventions were given could be varied systematically, to see if the effect was different at different ages. Attempts should also be made in analyses to detect interactions between types of persons and types of interventions.

The final issue that will be raised here is the extent to which interventions should be devised with an eye to implementation on a large scale. Should the interventions tested be chosen entirely on theoretical and prior research considerations or should they be limited to techniques that could feasibly be implemented as large-scale social policy? To a large extent, we have avoided this problem by not attempting to specify the techniques in great detail, just as we have not attempted to specify any other aspect of the design of the projects in great detail here. We are more concerned with laying down general principles. However, we believe that some version of all the interventions discussed here could be implemented in principle on a large scale.

Younger Population Cohorts

The major interventions we would propose for the younger population cohorts (between birth and age 12) are a "Head Start" type of preschool intellectual enrichment program such as that used by Schweinhart and Weikart (1980) and parent training of the type developed by Patterson (1980a). The Perry preschool program has already been discussed in Chapters 3 and 4. Briefly, the children attended a daily program that aimed to provide intellectual stimulation, to increase cognitive abilities, and to increase later school achievement. There were indications that the program was successful in reducing later delinquency and crime. The intellectual elements of the program could be supplemented by the caretakers providing warm attitudes, firm but kindly discipline, and desirable role models.

Patterson is well known for his careful observations of parent–child interaction. These showed that parents of antisocial children were deficient in their methods of child rearing. These parents failed to tell their children how they were expected to behave, failed to monitor the behavior to ensure that it was desirable, and failed to enforce rules promptly with appropriate rewards and penalties (Wilson, 1983). The parents of antisocial children used more punishment (such as scolding, shouting, or threatening), but failed to make it contingent on the child's behavior. Patterson then attempted to train these parents in effective child-rearing methods, namely, noticing what a child is doing, monitoring behavior over long periods, clearly stating house rules, making rewards and punishments contingent on behavior, and negotiating disagreements so that conflicts and crises did not escalate. His treatment has been shown to be effective in reducing child stealing over short periods in small-scale studies.

Another desirable intervention would be an elementary school program designed to improve school performance and motivation, if one could be found that had some empirical indications of success.

Older Population Cohorts

For the adolescent cohort, a program aimed at the peer group would be most desirable because delinquency between 12 and 18 is very much a group phenomenon and probably subject to peer facilitation. The most hopeful program in the literature is probably that by Feldman et al. (1983), which involved exposing antisocial juveniles to the influence of prosocial peer groups. This program would be worth replicating on a larger scale, although it might be difficult to set up in practice.

It might be more feasible to use a direct instruction or modeling approach such as that employed by Sarason (1978) with juvenile offenders. The subjects were taught such skills as how to resist peer pressures to engage in antisocial acts, how to delay gratification, and how to apply for a job. The approach used by Telch, Killen, McAlister, Perry, and Maccoby (1982) in successfully reducing adolescent smoking could also be built upon. They employed high school students to guide younger peers in developing counterarguing skills to resist peer pressures to smoke, using modeling and guided practice.

In view of the extensive evidence linking school failure and delinquency, it might also be worthwhile to try to develop a school program designed to improve performance and motivation (see Chapter 4). Possibly, some kind of recreational or community program designed to alleviate boredom by providing socially approved opportunities for excitement and risk taking could also be developed since a good deal of peer group delinquency seems to be linked to boredom, excitement seeking, and risk taking. Interestingly, an outward bound school program providing physical challenges and opportunities for risk taking seemed to be followed by lower recidivism than the regular Department of Youth Services treatment in a study by Kelly and Baer (1971) in Massachusetts, but this research was not well controlled. Another desirable program between the ages of 12 and 18 would be one aimed at decreasing drug use.

For the young adult cohort, the three obvious areas for intervention are employment, drug use, and helping to disengage from the peer group. In view of the link between unemployment and crime (Freeman, 1983), some kind of employment assistance program, if effective, should lead to a decrease in criminal behavior. Also, insofar as the decline in offending after age 20 seems to be linked to disengagement from the peer group (and settling down with a spouse or cohabitee), any measure that would facilitate this disengagement should decrease crime. As with the 12 to 18 age group, a drug program can also be recommended.

The Arrested Cohort

The interventions that can be studied with the arrested cohort depend on the degree of cooperation from criminal justice agencies. It is especially important to study the effectiveness of different dispositions, in comparison with no official action, if the authorities can be persuaded to assign offenders at random to different dispositions. One of the "dispositions" could be a diversion program, possibly based on the Binder and Newkirk (1977) study discussed in Chapter 3. Equally, it would be desirable to compare the effectiveness of juvenile and adult court, if juveniles could be waived to adult court at random. Another possible project would be a study of the effect on adult court processing of providing juvenile records, again presented to the adult court on a random basis. The justifications for these studies have been discussed in Chapter 4.

Depending on what appeared to be feasible, the definition of this cohort might have to be changed. For example, in comparing the effectiveness of juvenile and adult court, it might be better to follow up a sample of convicted rather than arrested juveniles. Similarly, in studying adult court processing, it might be better to define the sample according to court appearances at age 18 rather than arrests at age 15. However, insofar as the interest is in the transition from juvenile to adult court, it is important to document the natural history of criminal careers before the transition age is reached as well as after.

The Prison Cohort

The interventions that are possible with the prison cohort again depend to some extent on the degree of cooperation from official agencies. The programs can either be within the institution or after release. In regard to institutional interventions, one of the most interesting questions concerns the effect of length of time incarcerated on criminal careers (see Chapter 7). In investigating this, it would be desirable if some prisoners could be chosen at random for early release. Another intervention that could be studied is social-skills training. The theory underlying this is that the ability of people to achieve socially desirable goals such as material possessions, financial gain, vocational success, and peer status depends on their level of social skill, defined as their ability to elicit rewarding consequences in interpersonal interaction. The research of Sarason (1978) quoted in Chapter 3 was intended to teach social skills, and he found that his training led to a reduction in offending. Similarly, there are other studies (e.g., Spence, 1982) that yield enough guarded optimism about this procedure to make it worth investigating in more detail.

In regard to postprison interventions, the experiment of Rossi *et al.* (1980) suggests that an income-maintenance program might be effective in reducing offending if it does not include a disincentive to work. Some of the other experiments reviewed in Chapter 3 also suggest that practical assistance given to released prisoners (for example, in finding employment) could be effective in reducing offending. Therefore, both income maintenance and employment programs for ex-prisoners should be studied.

Subsidiary Issues

Preparatory Research

It is important that any longitudinal–experimental survey should be preceded by preparatory research and pilot work. This can include meta-analyses of existing literature and reanalyses of existing datasets. In addition, in the area under study, it is often worthwhile to carry out exploratory research, including case studies and unstructured interviews, retrospective searches of existing records, and possibly a cross-sectional survey of some of the age groups of interest. The point is that the longitudinal–experimental method involves a major commitment of resources, and careful preparation is necessary to reap all possible benefits from it.

Supplementary Studies

The major projects on the effects of interventions in longitudinal–experimental studies, described above, could be supplemented by smaller-scale studies. It would be especially useful to supplement the interview and record data by systematic observation, which is difficult to carry out on a large scale. Also, smaller-scale studies could involve more frequent measurement.

In the younger population cohorts, there could be detailed, extensive observation of parent–child interaction in the home, teacher–child interaction in the school, and of interaction between children in homes or schools or elsewhere. In the older population cohorts, there could be observation of peer group interaction and of interaction between spouses or cohabitees. In the arrested cohort, there could be observation of police–offender interactions and of exchanges in court, while in the prison cohort interactions between prisoners and guards, between prisoners and other prisoners, and even prison offenses could be observed systematically.

It might also be desirable to study biological factors in small-scale supplementary research. There are some indications of correlations between biological factors and measures of criminal behavior (e.g., Shah and Roth, 1974; Mednick and Volavka, 1980), but the precise causal linkages are not clear. As an example, offenders, and especially violent offenders, tend to have significantly low pulse rates (Wadsworth, 1976; Farrington, 1986b). The fact that it is difficult to measure many biological factors outside hospitals or institutions makes it hard to study them in the type of large-scale field research projects envisaged here. However, they are probably worth investigating in supplementary research that can be linked to the main project.

Some prevention programs could be implemented only on a small scale. For example, an attempt could be made to change interaction patterns in peer groups and make them less conducive to offending. In many ways, the model for these studies would be the work of Patterson (1980a) with families, beginning with careful, small-scale observations and continuing by trying to change interaction patterns. Smaller-scale studies could also be targeted on immediate situational influences on crime.

Quasi-Experimental Analyses

It would also be desirable to include quasi-experimental analyses in the major longitudinal–experimental studies, investigating the effects of events that are not under the control of the researcher. For example, in the younger population cohorts, the effects of a parent dying, leaving home, being arrested or convicted, or becoming unemployed could be studied, as could the effects of a sibling being arrested or convicted. In the older population cohorts, the effects of leaving school, getting a job, getting married, and becoming unemployed could be investigated. In the arrested or prison cohorts, the effects of nonrandomly assigned penalties or changes in the law could be studied, and the effects of prison riots or changes in prison rules or regimes. These analyses would normally be restricted to the cohorts that did not receive experimental interventions, to study events that occurred during the natural history of their criminal careers.

The Need for Replication

In the history of scientific endeavor, no single study, however well designed, can be conclusive. Every research project is limited to some extent by the particular setting in which it is conducted [see the section "Larger Experimental Units"], by the particular operational definitions of the theoretical variables, by the particular time period, and so on. In order to build up a solid body of knowledge, replication of key findings is vital. In the case of the proposed longitudinal–experimental studies, various kinds of replications are possible.

After the first series of cohorts has been followed up, it would be desirable to follow up a second series from the same areas and over the same age ranges. For example, after one cohort has been followed from birth to age 6, another can begin at birth. In the case of the older cohorts, a decision would have to be made about whether to continue following up the same cohort or whether to begin with a new cohort. For example, the second cohort followed up from 6 to 12 could either be a continuation of the first cohort followed up from birth to 6 or a new cohort selected at age 6. The best solution might be to have a combination of these two possibilities and to follow up those in the first cohort who had not been subject to the experimental manipulations (i.e., the controls) together with a newly selected group at the first age. This would make it possible to assess the effects of being studied, and it would reveal if there had been changes in the population in the area (e.g., due to immigration or emigration). It would also take advantage of the long-term developmental data on the first cohort while avoiding the effects of the experimental manipulations.

In the new series of cohorts, it would be possible to take account of changes in theories, methods of research and measurement, and policy concerns during the first series, and also to build on the results obtained in the first series. In addition, the new series of cohorts would permit the separation of aging and period effects. Comparisons between one age in the first series and the same age in the second would give some indication of changes over the period, while comparisons between changes between two ages in the first series and changes between the same two ages in the second would give some indication about changes with age.

The second series of cohorts would have to be planned in light of the results of the first series, aiming for cumulative knowledge. A cheaper and quicker way of separating aging and period effects would be to carry out a cross-sectional survey of a sample aged from birth to 24 at the start of the first series and to repeat this at the end. However, this would not have the other advantages of the second series in building on and extending the results of the first series and in taking account of changes in theories, methods, and policy concerns.

In addition to replication with new cohorts in the same area, it would of course be desirable to study how far the findings could be replicated in other areas, with other operational definitions of the interventions and other criminal justice systems. In addition, as noted earlier, it would be useful to establish how far interventions had similar impacts in rural (as opposed to urban) areas or with older persons. These are probably longer-term goals.

Larger Experimental Units

It would also be useful to supplement the major longitudinal–experimental studies of individuals with similar studies based on larger units, where possible. In particular, it would be desirable to carry out research in the areas from which the population cohorts are drawn and in the prisons from which the prison cohort is drawn. The aim would be to study the effect of an experimentally induced change in one area compared with a control area that did not experience the change. An example of this method would be the research by Buikhuisen (1974) quoted in Chapter 3. However, the aim would also be to compare changes in the area with data collected from individuals in the area as part of the longitudinal–experimental study and, hence, to link individual criminal careers with community crime careers.

The projects could investigate the effects of experimenter-controlled changes in the areas (such as providing more facilities for youth, changing police patrolling strategies, or introducing community projects such as Block Watch aimed at decreasing situational crime opportunities) on area measures such as the observed amount of vandalism or the level of victim-reported crime and on the individuals in the major studies. Another project could study the effects of experimenter-controlled changes in a prison (such as the introduction of partitions in dormitories to increase perceived privacy) on prison measures such as the amount of damage and on the prisoners in the major longitudinal–experimental study. The manipulations that could be introduced in the areas or the prisons would depend on the degree of cooperation from official agencies, of course.

It would also be desirable to conduct some supplementary studies based on peer groups or families as units. In the case of peer groups, youths should be asked to nominate their friends, and changes in peer group associations could be linked to changes in delinquent behavior. The key issue is the extent to which newly developing associations with deviant peers facilitate newly developing delinquent behavior. Detailed attempts could be made to link up individual criminal careers into group careers.

As mentioned earlier, in studying larger units, one of the most pressing needs is to link the individual criminal career to the social context—the area, the school, neighborhood social service agencies, employment opportunities, and so on. Understanding individual criminal careers is likely to be enhanced by knowledge of the institutional contexts in which they are located.

Problems of Implementation

Organizing the Research Program

In view of the difficulty of mounting the major longitudinal–experimental projects proposed here, it is important that they be planned with the research community in mind. The aim should be to build a large and growing database to serve the needs of a variety of people in primary and secondary analyses. The marginal costs of extra data collection might not be very great in comparison with the long-term benefits to the research community. This is one reason, in addition to the versatility of deviant behavior, for attempting to measure a wide variety of deviant acts or social problems as well as strictly criminal behavior. If drug use, heavy drinking, heavy gambling, child abuse, family violence, unemployment, sexual prosmiscuity, reckless driving (and so on) are all measured in the proposed longitudinal–experimental projects, then researchers in all these disparate fields can make use of the resulting datasets and estimate the effects of the interventions on many different kinds of social problems. This is one way to justify the cost of the proposed projects.

The two alternative methods of organizing the project involve either (a) a principal investigator taking primary responsibility for the design, data collection, and analysis, guided by a steering committee or (b) a consortium of investigators taking primary responsibility for the design and analysis and contracting out the data collection to an agency such as the U.S. Bureau of the Census or the Survey Research Center of the University of Michigan. The two models have complementary advantages and disadvantages. Some advantages of the principal-investigator model are that there can be closer quality control over and understanding of the data collection and that decisions can be made more speedily. Also, the energizing drive and enthusiasm of a strong, committed leader may be necessary to carry through a long and complex project to a successful conclusion. Some advantages of the consortium model follow from the greater breadth of multidisciplinary perspectives and expertise involved in the design and analysis and the more comprehensive range of data collected and hypotheses tested. It might prove more attractive to funding agencies to invest a large amount of money in a consortium rather than a single center. Indeed, a consortium of funding agencies may be needed to finance a large-scale project.

In practice, it might be unnecessary to choose between the two alternatives because there may be little difference between a principal investigator advised by a powerful, committed, and involved steering group, and a consortium led by a powerful, decisive chairperson. In either case, it is desirable to ensure that the data collected are made available to the research community in a timely fashion and to secure a long-term commitment to the program by the researchers.

The major practical problems center on obtaining a long-term guarantee of funding and ensuring the continuity of the research program. It may be that a foundation could provide more stable funding than a federal agency because a foundation might be able to work to a longer time horizon. As already mentioned, it would be desirable to choose the location of the research according to criteria such as the mobility of the population, the adequacy of available records, the cooperativeness of the community, and the cooperativeness of official agencies in allowing access to records, in helping to locate subjects, and in allowing randomized experiments. The first research project to be carried out should be designed to identify the best locations for a longitudinal–experimental study. From the viewpoint of justifying the study in terms of public policy importance, it is important to treat crime problems in the inner city as a primary target.

There may be practical difficulties in arranging for experimental interventions because criminal justice professionals may be unwilling to allow randomization. There may also be ethical and legal problems of denying treatment to certain persons. These kinds of problems have been discussed by Farrington (1983c). It would be desirable to use the term "equal probability assignment" rather than "random assignment" because of the association of the word "random" with "arbitrary" (see Garner, 1977).

How Much Will It Cost?

It is impossible to derive an accurate estimate of the likely cost of a longitudinal–experimental project such as that proposed here without going into much more detail about the precise nature of the project. However, we will attempt a rough order of magnitude estimate.

One of the most expensive options would involve some 6,000 face-to-face interviews per year for seven years (e.g., ages 6 to 12) in an area, plus preparatory research, experimental manipulations, and subsidiary studies. This assumes that each person in the 6 cohorts has only one face-to-face interview per year and that data from other persons is collected by other means (e.g., telephone interviews or self-completed questionnaires). The cost of the project could be cut down by replacing some of the face-to-face interviews by telephone interviews. For example, if there were face-to-face interviews only at the start, in the middle, and at the end of the period, and telephone interviews in the intervening years, the total cost of the project might be roughly one-third less.

The most comparable ongoing survey is probably that directed by Elliott (e.g., Elliott et al., 1983). For about 1,700 face-to-face interviews throughout the United States in a year, plus searches of police records, the price was $400,000 in direct costs per year (including developing the instrument, pretesting, interviewer training, interviewing, data processing, and data analysis; Elliott, personal communication). This could be cut down to about $300,000 per year by using telephone interviews. The cost of experimental manipulations is hard to quantify, but a ball-park figure might be $200,000 per year. To all of these direct costs must be added indirect costs of about 50%.

Bearing in mind the fact that the proposed study will be conducted only in one SMSA, but that it will involve more extensive data collection than in the Elliott survey, it might be possible to carry out some variant of the proposed longitudinal–experimental project for about $1,000,000 per year.

If this cost seems high, it should be compared with criminal justice system costs. For example, according to Rossi *et al.* (1980), the average cost of keeping their ex-prisoners in prison was $13,500 per person per year. At that rate, $1,000,000 only equates to 74 prisoners for one year. Therefore, $1,000,000 spent on research would pay for itself if it prevented the equivalent of 74 person-years of imprisonment; and this does not count the cost of the crimes to the victims or the community or the cost of police or court processing. Also, as Berk, Boruch, Chambers, Rossi, and Witte (1985) have argued, there are costs in not experimenting if this means that a great deal of money is spent on ineffective programs.

Conclusions

We have outlined a number of longitudinal–experimental projects in this chapter that we believe would greatly advance our knowledge about the causes, prevention, and treatment of crime. These projects aim to provide information about the development of criminal careers and about the effects of interventions on these careers. Apart from the longitudinal–experimental method, these projects are unique in their attempt to link data from different surveys to build up a complete picture of the criminal career.

We have not tried to specify the projects in detail. Our examples are meant to be illustrative, not prescriptive. Nor can we claim that they will throw light on every topic of current interest in crime and justice. Like much previous research, they are targeted on crimes by young persons in large cities. We also cannot claim that our proposed interventions are new. However, by and large, their choice can be justified empirically, and there is some reason to be cautiously confident that they will have the intended effects on criminal behavior. At the very least, the projects would yield an outstandingly important data resource that could be used for many years to test a variety of hypotheses, including some not foreseen at the beginning.

We believe that now is the time to mount one or more major longitudinal–experimental studies. The major investment of resources would be justified by the significant advancement of knowledge, which in due course should contribute to a significant reduction in serious and frequent offending. That would be in everyone's interest.

References

Adams, S.
   1970   "The PICO project." Pp. 548–561 in N. Johnston, L. Savitz, and M.E. Wolfgang
          (eds.). The Sociology of Punishment and Correction. New York: Wiley.
Ageton, S.S.
   1983   "The dynamics of female delinquency, 1976–1980." Criminology 21:555–584.
Alexander, J.F and B.V. Parsons
   1973   "Short-term behavioral intervention with delinquent families: impact on family
          process and recidivism." Journal of Abnormal Psychology 81:219–225.
Allen, F.A.
   1981   The Decline of the Rehabilitative Ideal. New Haven, CT: Yale University Press.
Andenaes, J.
   1977   "The general preventive effects of punishment." Pp. 20–53 in L. Radzinowicz
          and M. Wolfgang (eds). Crime and Justice, Volume II. Revised edition. New
          York: Basic Books, Inc.
Annis, H.M.
   1979   "Group treatment of incarcerated offenders with alcohol and drug problems: a
          controlled evaluation." Canadian Journal of Criminology 21:3–15.
Ares, C.E., A. Rankin and H. Sturz
   1963   "The Manhattan bail project." New York University Law Review 38:67–92.
Attorney General's Task Force on Family Violence
   1984   (September) Final Report. Washington, D.C.: U.S. Dept. of Justice.
Bachman, J.G., P.M. O'Malley and J. Johnston
   1978   Youth in Transition. Volume 6. Ann Arbor, MI: University of Michigan Institute
          for Social Research.
Baker, S.H. and S. Sadd
   1981   Diversion of Felony Arrests. Washington, D.C.: National Institute of Law
          Enforcement and Criminal Justice.
Baldwin, J.
   1979   "Ecological and areal studies in Great Britain and the United States." Pp. 29–66
          in N. Morris and M. Tonry (eds.). Crime and Justice: An Annual Review of
          Research. Volume 1. Chicago: University of Chicago Press.
Ball, J.C., L. Rosen, J.A. Flueck and D.N. Nurco
   1981   "The criminality of heroin addicts: when addicted and when off opiates. Pp.
          39–65 in J.A. Inciardi (ed.). The Drugs–Crime Connection. Beverly Hills, CA:
          Sage.

Barnett, A. and A. Lofaso
  1985 "Selective incapacitative and the Philadelphia cohort data." Journal of Quantitative Criminology 1:3–36.

Baron, R. and F. Feeney
  1976 Juvenile Diversion Through Family Counseling. Washington, D.C.: National Institute of Law Enforcement and Criminal Justice.

Baron, R., F. Feeney and W. Thornton
  1973 "Preventing delinquency through diversion." Federal Probation 37(1):13–18.

Belsky, J.
  1980 "Child maltreatment: an ecological integration." American Psychologist 35:320–335.
  1981 "Early human experience: a family perspective." Developmental Psychology 17:3–23.

Berg, I., M. Costerdine, R. Hullin, R. McGuire and S. Tyrer
  1978 "The effect of two randomly allocated court procedures on truancy." British Journal of Criminology 18:232–244.

Berg, I., R. Hullin and R. McGuire
  1979 "A randomly controlled trial of two court procedures in truancy." Pp. 143–151 in D.P. Farrington, K. Hawkins and S.M. Lloyd-Bostock (eds.). Psychology, Law and Legal Processes. London: Macmillan.

Berk, R.A., R.F. Boruch, D.L. Chambers, P.H. Rossi and A.D. Witte
  1985 "Social policy experimentation: a position paper." Evaluation Review 9:387–429.

Berntsen, K. and K.O. Christiansen
  1965 "A resocialization experiment with short-term offenders." Pp. 35–54 in K.O. Christiansen (ed.). Scandinavian Studies in Criminology. Volume 1. London: Tavistock.

Berrueta-Clement, J.R., L.J. Schweinhart, W.S. Barnett, A.S. Epstein and D.P. Weikart
  1984 Changed Lives. Ypsilanti, MI: High/Scope.

Binder, A.
  1978 Pretrial Intervention and Diversion Project: Final Report. Unpublished manuscript.

Binder, A., J. Monahan and M. Newkirk
  1976 "Diversion from the juvenile justice system and the prevention of delinquency." Pp. 131–140 in J. Monahan (ed.). Community Mental Health and the Criminal Justice System. New York: Pergamon.

Binder, A. and M. Newkirk
  1977 "A program to extend police service capability." Crime Prevention Review 4:26–32.

Black, D.J. and A.J. Reiss, Jr.
  1970 "Police control of juveniles." American Sociological Review 35:63–77.

Blumstein, A. and J. Cohen
  1979 "Estimation of individual crime rates from arrest records." Journal of Criminal Law and Criminology 70:561–585.

Blumstein, A., J. Cohen and P. Hsieh
  1982 "The duration of adult criminal careers." Final Report to National Institute of Justice. Washington, D.C.: National Institute of Justice.

Blumstein, A., J. Cohen and D. Nagin (eds.)
  1978 Deterrence and Incapacitation: Estimating the Effects of Criminal Sanctions on Crime Rates. Washington, D.C.: National Academy of Sciences.

Blumstein, A., D.P. Farrington and S. Moitra
  1985 "Delinquency careers: innocents, desisters, and persisters." Pp. 187–219 in M. Tonry and N. Morris (eds.). Crime and Justice: An Annual Review of Research. Volume 6. Chicago: University of Chicago Press.

Blumstein, A. and S. Moitra
  1980 "The identification of 'career criminals' from 'chronic offenders' in a cohort." Law and Policy Quarterly 2:321–334.

Bohman, M.
  1978 "Some genetic aspects of alcoholism and criminality." Archives of General Psychiatry 35:269–276.

Boland, B. and J.Q. Wilson
  1978 "Age, crime, and punishment." The Public Interest 51:22–34.

Botein, B.
  1965 "The Manhattan bail project: its impact on criminology and the criminal law processes." Texas Law Review 43:319–331.

Bowker L.
  1977 Prisoner Subcultures. Lexington, MA: D.C. Heath.

Boyanowsky, E.O. and C.T. Griffiths
  1982 "Weapons and eye contact as instigators and inhibitors of aggressive arousal in police–citizen interaction." Journal of Applied Social Psychology 12:398–407.

Brody, S.R.
  1976 The Effectiveness of Sentencing. London: Her Majesty's Stationery Office.

Buckle, A. and D.P. Farrington
  1984 "An observational study of shoplifting." British Journal of Criminology 24:63–73.

Buikhuisen, W.
  1974 "General deterrence: research and theory." Abstracts in Criminology and Penology 14:285–298.

Bureau of Justice Statistics
  1983 Report to the Nation on Crime and Justice: The Data. Washington, D.C.: U.S. Department of Justice.
  1984a The Severity of Crime. Washington, D.C.: U.S. Department of Justice.
  1984b Prisoners in 1983. Washington, D.C.: U.S. Department of Justice.

Bursik, R.J.
  1980 "The dynamics of specialization in juvenile offenses." Social Forces 58:851–864.

Bursik, R.J. and J. Webb
  1982 "Community change and patterns of delinquency." American Journal of Sociology 88:24–42.

Byles, J.A. and A. Maurice
  1979 "The juvenile services project: an experiment in delinquency control." Canadian Journal of Criminology 21:155–165.

Cadoret, R.J. and C. Cain
  1980 "Sex differences as predictors of antisocial behavior in adoptees." Archives of General Psychiatry 37:1171–1175.

Campbell, D.T. and H.L. Ross
  1968 "The Connecticut crackdown on speeding." Law and Society Review 3:33–53.

Campbell, D.T. and J.C. Stanley
  1966 Experimental and Quasi-Experimental Designs for Research. Chicago: Rand McNally.

Carroll, L.
  1974   Hacks, Blacks and Cons. Lexington, MA: Heath.
Cattell, R.B.
  1982   The Inheritance of Personality and Ability: Research Methods and Findings.
         New York: Academic Press.
Chaiken, J.M. and M.R. Chaiken
  1982   Varieties of Criminal Behavior. Santa Monica, CA: Rand.
Chess, S. and A. Thomas
  1984   Origins and Evolution of Behavior Disorders. New York: Brunner/Mazel.
Christiansen, K.O.
  1968   "Threshold of tolerance in various population groups illustrated by results from
         Danish criminological twin study." Pp. 107–116 in A.V.S. De Reuck and R.
         Porter (eds.). The Mentally Abnormal Offender. London: Churchill.
  1974   "Seriousness of criminality and concordance among Danish twins." Pp. 63–77 in
         R. Hood (ed.). Crime, Criminology, and Public Policy. London: Heinemann.
Clarke, S.H.
  1974   "Getting 'em out of circulation: does incarceration of juvenile offenders reduce
         crime?" Journal of Criminal Law and Criminology 65:528–535.
  1975   "Some implications for North Carolina of recent research in juvenile delin-
         quency." Journal of Research in Crime and Delinquency 12:51–60.
Clemmer, D.
  1940   The Prison Community. New York: Holt, Rinehart, and Winston.
Cline, H.F.
  1980   "Criminal behavior over the life span." Pp. 641–674 in O.G. Brim and J. Kagan
         (eds.). Constancy and Change in Human Development. Cambridge, MA: Har-
         vard University Press.
Cloninger, C.R., M. Bohman and S. Sigvardsson
  1981   "Inheritance of alcohol abuse." Archives of General Psychiatry 38:861–868.
Cloward, R.A. and L.E. Ohlin
  1960   Delinquency and Opportunity. New York: Free Press.
Cohen, A.K.
  1955   Delinquent Boys. Glencoe, IL: Free Press.
Cohen, J.
  1983a "Incapacitation as a strategy for crime control: possibilities and pitfalls." Pp.
         1–84 in M. Tonry and N. Morris (eds.). Crime and Justice: An Annual Review
         of Research. Volume 5. Chicago: University of Chicago Press.
  1983b Incapacitating Criminals: Recent Research Findings of Justice. Washington,
         D.C.: U.S. Government Printing Office.
Collins, J.J.
  1981   "Alcohol careers and criminal careers." Pp. 152–206 in J.J. Collins (ed.). Drink-
         ing and Crime. New York: Guilford Press.
Consortium for Longitudinal Studies
  1983   As the Twig is Bent . . . Lasting Effects of Preschool Programs. Hillsdale, NJ:
         Lawrence Erlbaum.
Cook, T.D. and D.T. Campbell
  1979   Quasi-experimentation. Chicago: Rand McNally.
Cooley, C.H.
  1902   Human Nature and the Social Order. New York: Scribner.

Cornish, D.B. and R.V.G. Clarke
  1975 Residential Treatment and its Effects on Delinquency. London: Her Majesty's
        Stationery Office.
Dalgard, O.S. and E. Kringlen
  1976 "A Norwegian twin study of criminality." British Journal of Criminology
        16:213–232.
Douglas, J.W.B.
  1970 "Discussion." Pp. 86–89 in E.H. Hare and J.K. Wing (eds.). Psychiatric
        Epidemiology. London: Oxford University Press.
Douglas, J.W.B., J.M. Ross and H.R. Simpson
  1968 All Our Future. London: Peter Davies.
Dunford, F.W., D.W. Osgood and H.F. Weichselbaum
  1982 National Evaluation of Diversion Projects. Washington, D.C.: National Institute
        of Juvenile Justice and Delinquency Prevention.
Dunford, F.W. and D.S. Elliott
  1984 "Identifying career offenders using self-reported data." Journal of Research in
        Crime and Delinquency 21:57–86.
Dunlop, A.B.
  1974 The Approved School Experience. London: Her Majesty's Stationery Office.
Edmonds, R.R. and J.R. Frederikson
  1978 Search for Effective Schools: The Identification and Analysis of City Schools
        That Are Instructionally Effective for Poor Children. Cambridge, MA: Harvard
        University Center for Urban Studies.
Ekland-Olson, S., J. Lieb and L. Zurcher
  1984 "The paradoxical impact of criminological sanctions: some microstructural find-
        ings." Law and Society Review 18:159–178.
Elliott, D.S., S.S. Ageton and R.J. Canter
  1979 "An integrated theoretical perspective on delinquent behavior." Journal of
        Research in Crime and Delinquency 16:3–27.
Elliott, D.S., S.S. Ageton, D. Huizinga, B.A. Knowles and R.J. Canter
  1983 The Prevalence and Incidence of Delinquent Behavior: 1976–1980. Boulder,
        CO: Behavioral Research Institute.
Elliott, D.S. and D. Huizinga
  1983 "Social class and delinquent behavior in a national youth panel: 1976–1980."
        Criminology 21:149–177.
  1984 The Relationship Between Delinquent Behavior and ADM Problems. Boulder,
        CO: Behavioral Research Institute.
Elliott, D.S., D. Huizinga and S.S. Ageton
  1985 Explaining Delinquency and Drug Use. Beverly Hills, CA: Sage.
Elliott, D.S., B.A. Knowles and R.J. Canter
  1981 The Epidemiology of Delinquent Behavior and Drug Use Among American
        Adolescents. Boulder, CO: Behavioral Research Institute.
Elliott, D.S. and H.L. Voss
  1974 Delinquency and Dropout. Lexington, MA: Heath.
Empey, L.T. and M.L. Erickson
  1972 The Provo Experiment. Lexington, MA: Heath.
Empey, L.T. and S.G. Lubeck
  1971 The Silverlake Experiment. Chicago: Aldine.

Ericson, R.V.

   1977   "Social distance and reaction to criminality." British Journal of Criminology 17:16–29.

Eron, L.D.

   1982   (August) "The consistency of aggressive behavior across time and situations." Paper presented at the Annual Convention of the American Psychological Association, Anaheim, CA.

Eysenck, H.J.

   1964   Crime and Personality. London: Routledge and Kegan Paul.

Farrington, D.P.

   1972   "Delinquency begins at home." New Society 21:495–497.

   1973   "Self-reports of deviant behavior: predictive and stable?" Journal of Criminal Law and Criminology 64:99–110.

   1977   "The effects of public labeling." British Journal of Criminology 17:112–125.

   1978   "The family backgrounds of aggressive youths." Pp. 73–93 in L. Hersov, M. Berger and D. Shaffer (eds.). Aggression and Antisocial Behavior in Childhood and Adolescence. Oxford: Pergamon.

   1979a "Delinquent behavior modification in the natural environment." British Journal of Criminology 19:353–372.

   1979b "Experiments on deviance with special reference to dishonesty." Pp. 207–252 in L. Berkowitz (ed.). Advances in Experimental Social Psychology. volume 12. New York: Academic Press.

   1979c "Longitudinal research on crime and delinquency." Pp. 289–348 in N. Morris and M. Tonry (eds.). Crime and Justice: An Annual Review of Research. Volume 1. Chicago: University of Chicago Press.

   1981   Prevention of juvenile delinquency: an introduction. Pp. 5–10 in Prevention of Juvenile Delinquency: The Role of Institutions of Socialization in a Changing Society. Fourteenth Criminological Research Conference, Stasbourg, France: Council of Europe.

   1983a Further Analyses of a Longitudinal Survey of Crime and Delinquency. Final Report to National Institute of Justice. Washington, D.C.: National Institute of Justice.

   1983b "Offending from 10 to 25 years of age." Pp. 17–37 in K.T. Van Dusen and S.A. Mednick (eds.). Prospective Studies of Crime and Delinquency. Boston: Kluwer-Nijhoff.

   1983c "Randomized experiments on crime and justice." Pp. 257–308 in M. Tonry and N. Morris (eds). Crime and Justice: An Annual Review of Research. Volume 4. Chicago: University of Chicago Press.

   1985   "Delinquency prevention in the 1980s." Journal of Adolescence 8:3–16.

   1986a "Age and crime." Pp. 29–90 in M. Tonry and N. Morris (eds.). Crime and Justice: An Annual Review of Research. Volume 7. Chicago: University of Chicago Press, in press.

   1986b "Implications of biological findings for criminological research." In S.A. Mednick and T.E. Moffitt (eds.). The New Biocriminology. New York: Cambridge University Press, in press.

   1986c "Stepping stones to adult criminal careers." Pp. 359–384 in D. Olweus, J. Block and M.R. Yarrow (eds.). Development of Antisocial and Prosocial Behavior. New York: Academic Press.

Farrington, D.P. and E.A. Dowds
  1985 "Disentangling criminal behavior and police reaction." Pp. 41–72 in D.P. Far-
    rington and J. Gunn (eds.). Reactions to Crime: The Public, The Police, Courts,
    and Prisons. Chichester, England: Wiley.
Farrington, D.P. and C.P. Nuttall
  1980 "Prison size, overcrowding, prison violence, and recidivism." Journal of Crimi-
    nal Justice 8:221–231.
Farrington, D.P., S.G. Osborn and D.J. West
  1978 "The persistence of labeling effects." British Journal of Criminology 18:277–284.
Farrington, D.P. and R. Tarling
  1985 "Criminological prediction: an introduction." Pp. 2–33 in D.P. Farrington and
    R. Tarling (eds.). Prediction in Criminology. Albany, NY: State University of
    New York Press.
Farrington, D.P. and D.J. West
  1981 "The Cambridge study in delinquent development." Pp. 137–145 in S.A. Med-
    nick and A.E. Baert (eds.). Prospective Longitudinal Research. Oxford: Oxford
    University Press.
Feld, B.C.
  1977 Neutralizing Inmate Violence: Juvenile Offenders in Institutions. Cambridge:
    Ballinger.
  1981 "Legislative politics toward the serious juvenile offender: on the virtues of auto-
    matic adulthood." Crime and Delinquency 27:497–521.
Feldhusen, J.F., F.M. Aversano and J.R. Thurston
  1976 "Prediction of youth contacts with law enforcement agencies." Criminal Justice
    and Behavior 3:235–253.
Feldhusen, J.F., J.R. Thurston and J.J. Benning
  1973 "A longitudinal study of delinquency and other aspects of children's behavior."
    International Journal of Criminology and Penology 1:341–351.
Feldman, R.A., T.E. Caplinger and J.S. Wodarski
  1983 The St. Louis Conundrum. Englewood Cliffs, NJ: Prentice-Hall.
Fienberg, S.E., K. Larntz and A.J. Reiss
  1976 "Redesigning the Kansas City preventive patrol experiment." Evaluation
    3:124–131.
Finckenauer, J.O.
  1982 Scared Straight. Englewood Cliffs, NJ: Prentice-Hall.
Fischer, D.G.
  1983 "Parental supervision and delinquency." Perceptual and Motor Skills
    56:635–640.
Fishman, S. and A.S. Alissi
  1979 "Strengthening families as natural support systems for offenders." Federal Pro-
    bation 43(3):16–21.
Flanagan, T.J.
  1980 "The pains of long-term imprisonment." British Journal of Criminology
    20:148–167.
Fo, W.S.O. and C.R. O'Donnell
  1974 "The buddy system: relationship and contingency conditions in a community
    intervention program for youth with nonprofessionals as behavior change
    agents." Journal of Consulting and Clinical Psychology 42:163–169.

1975   "The buddy system: effect of community intervention on delinquent offenses."
        Behavior Therapy 6:522–524.

Folkard, M., D.E. Smith and D.D. Smith
1976   IMPACT. Volume 2. London: Her Majesty's Stationery Office.

Fowles, A.J.
1978   Prison Welfare. London: Her Majesty's Stationery Office.

Freeman, R.B.
1983   "Crime and unemployment." Pp. 89–106 in J.Q. Wilson (ed.). Crime and Public
        Policy. San Francisco, CA: Institute for Contemporary Studies.

Gaes, G.G.
1985   "The effects of overcrowding in prison." Pp. 95–146 in M. Tonry and N. Morris
        (ed.). Crime and Justice: An Annual Review of Research. Volume 6. Chicago:
        University of Chicago Press.

Garabedian, P.G.
1963   "Social roles and processes of socialization in the prison community." Social
        Problems 11:139–152.

Garbarino, J. and M.C. Plantz
1984   (April) "Child maltreatment and juvenile delinquency: what are the links?"
        Paper presented at symposium on Child Abuse and Juvenile Delinquency,
        Racine, WI.

Garfinkel, H.
1956   "Conditions of successful degradation ceremonies." American Journal of Sociol-
        ogy 61:420–424.

Garner, J.H.
1977   "The role of Congress in program evaluation: three examples in criminal
        justice." Prison Journal 57:3–12.

Gault, V.
1967   in re, 387 U.S. 1.

Gibbens, T.C.N.
1984   "Borstal boys after 25 years." British Journal of Criminology 24:49–62.

Gibbs, J.P.
1975   Crime, Punishment, and Deterrence. New York: Elsevier.

Glaser, D.
1964   The Effectiveness of a Prison and Parole System. Indianapolis, IN: Bobbs-
        Merrill.

1978   Crime in our Changing Society. New York: Holt, Rinehart, and Winston.

Glueck, S. and E.T. Glueck
1930   Five Hundred Criminal Careers. New York: Knopf.

1934   One Thousand Juvenile Delinquents. Cambridge, MA: Harvard University
        Press.

1937   Later Criminal Careers. New York: Commonwealth Fund.

1940   Juvenile Delinquents Grown Up. New York: Commonwealth Fund.

1943   Criminal Careers in Retrospect. New York: Commonwealth Fund.

1950   Unraveling Juvenile Delinquency. Cambridge, MA: Harvard University Press.

1968   Delinquents and Non-Delinquents in Perspective. Cambridge, MA: Harvard
        University Press.

Gold, M.
1970   Delinquent Behavior in an American City. Belmont, CA: Brooks/Cole.

Gold, M. and D.J. Reimer
  1975 "Changing patterns of delinquent behavior among Americans 13 through 16 years old: 1967–1972." Crime and Delinquency Literature 7:483–517.
Gold, M. and J.R. Williams
  1969 "National study of the aftermath of apprehension." Prospectus: A Journal of Law Reform 3:3–12.
Goodstein, L.
  1976 "Inmate adjustment to prison and the transition to community life." Journal of Research in Crime and Delinquency 16:246–272.
Gordon, R.A.
  1976 "Prevalence: the rare datum in delinquency measurement and its implications for the theory of delinquency." Pp. 201–284 in M.W. Klein (ed.). The Juvenile Justice System. Beverly Hills, CA: Sage.
Graham, F.
  1981 "Probability of detection and institutional vandalism." British Journal of Criminology 21:361–365.
Greenberg, D.F. (ed.)
  1981 Crime and Capitalism: Readings in Marxist Criminology. Palo Alto, CA: Mayfield.
Greenwood, P.W.
  1980 "Career criminal prosecution." Journal of Criminal Law and Criminology 71:85–88.
Greenwood, P.W. and A. Abrahamse
  1982 Selective Incapacitation. Santa Monica, CA: Rand.
Greenwood, P.W., J. Petersilia and F.E. Zimring
  1980 Age, Crime, and Sanctions: The Transition from Juvenile to Adult Court. Santa Monica, CA: Rand.
Guttridge, P., W.F. Gabrielli, S.A. Mednick and K.T. Van Dusen
  1983 "Criminal violence in a birth cohort." Pp. 211–224 in K.T. Van Dusen and S.A. Mednick (eds.). Prospective Studies of Crime and Delinquency. Boston: Kluwer-Nijhoff.
Hamparian, D.M., R. Schuster, S. Dinitz and J.P. Conrad
  1978 The Violent Few. Lexington, MA: Heath.
Hamparian, D.M., L.K. Estep, S.M. Muntean, R.R. Priestino, R.G. Swisher, P.L. Wallace and J.L. White
  1982 Youth in Adult Courts: Between Two Worlds. Columbus, OH: Academy for Contemporary Problems.
Handler, J.F. and J. Zatz (eds.)
  1982 Neither Angels Nor Thieves: Studies in Deinstitutionalization of Status Offenders. Washington, D.C.: National Academy Press.
Haney, C., C. Banks and P. Zimbardo
  1973 "Interpersonal dynamics in a simulated prison." International Journal of Criminology and Penology 1:69–97.
Hartl, E.M., E.P. Monnelly and R.D. Elderkin
  1982 Physique and Delinquent Behavior. New York: Academic Press.
Hathaway, S.R. and E.D. Monachesi
  1957 "The personalities of pre-delinquent boys." Journal of Criminal Law, Criminology, and Police Science 48:149–163.

1963   Adolescent Personality and Behavior. Minneapolis, MN: University of Minnesota Press.

Hathaway, S.R., E.D. Monachesi and L.A. Young
1960   "Delinquency rates and personality." Journal of Criminal Law, Criminology, and Police Science 50:433–440.

Hathaway, S.R., P.C. Reynolds and E.D. Monachesi
1969   "Follow-up of the later careers and lives of 1,000 boys who dropped out of high school." Journal of Consulting and Clinical Psychology 33:370–380.

Havighurst, R.J., P.H. Bowman, G.P. Liddle, C.V. Matthews and J.V. Pierce
1962   Growing Up in River City. New York: Wiley.

Hawkins, J.D., C.H. Cassidy, N.B. Light and C.A. Miller
1977   "Interpreting official records as indicators of recidivism in evaluating delinquency prevention programs." Criminology 15:397–424.

Hindelang, M.J.
1971   "Age, sex, and the versatility of delinquent involvements." Social Problems 18:522–535.

Hindelang, M.J., T. Hirschi and J.G. Weis
1981   Measuring Delinquency. Beverly Hills, CA: Sage.

Hirschi, T.
1969   Causes of Delinquency. Berkeley, CA: University of California Press.
1980   "Labelling theory and juvenile delinquency: an assessment of the evidence." Pp. 271–302 in W.R. Gove (ed.). The Labelling of Deviance: Evaluating a Perspective. Beverly Hills, CA: Sage.

Hirschi, T. and M. Gottfredson
1983   "Age and the explanation of crime." American Journal of Sociology 89:552–584.

Hogh, E. and P. Wolf
1981   "Project Metropolitan: a longitudinal study of 12,270 boys from the metropolitan area of Copenhagen, Denmark (1953–77)." Pp. 99–103 in S.A. Mednick and A.E. Baert (eds.). Prospective Longitudinal Research. Oxford: Oxford University Press.

Holden, R.T.
1983   "Rehabilitative sanctions for drunk driving: an experimental evaluation." Journal of Research in Crime and Delinquency 20:55–72.

Holt, N. and D. Miller
1972   (January) Explorations in Inmate–Family Relationships. Sacramento, CA: California Department of Corrections, Report Number 46.

Home Office
1983   Criminal Statistics, England and Wales, 1982. London: Her Majesty's Stationary Office.
1985   (July) Criminal Careers of Those Born in 1953, 1958, and 1963. London: Home Office Statistical Bulletin.

Homer, E.
1979   "Inmate–family ties: desirable but difficult." Federal Probation 43(1):47–52.

Hood, R. and R. Sparks
1970   Key Issues in Criminology. London: Weidenfeld and Nicolson.

Hunner, R.H. and Y.E. Walker (eds.)
1981   Exploring the Relationship Between Child Abuse and Delinquency. Montclair, NJ: Allanheld, Osmun.

Irwin, J.
 1970 The Felon. Englewood Cliffs, NJ: Prentice-Hall.
 1980 Prisons in Turmoil. Boston: Little, Brown.
Irwin, J. and D. Cressey
 1962 "Thieves, convicts, and the inmate culture." Social Problems 10:142–155.
Jacobs, J.B.
 1977a Stateville, The Penitentiary in a Mass Society. Chicago: University of Chicago
        Press.
 1977b "Street gangs behind bars." Pp. 186–203 in R.M. Carter, D. Glaser and L.T.
        Wilkins (eds.). Correctional Institutions. Philadelphia: Lippincott.
 1979 "Race relations and the prisoner subculture." Pp. 1–27 in N. Morris and M.
        Tonry (eds.). Crime and Justice: An Annual Review of Research. Vol. 1.
        Chicago: University of Chicago Press.
Jacobs, J.B., R. McGahey and R. Minion
 1984 "Ex-offender employment, recidivism and manpower policy: CETA, TJTC, and
        future initiatives." Crime and Delinquency 30:486–506.
Janson, C.G.
 1981 "Project Metropolitan: a longitudinal study of a Stockholm cohort." Pp. 93–99
        in S.A. Mednick and A.E. Baert (eds.). Prospective Longitudinal Research.
        Oxford: Oxford University Press.
Jensen, G.F.
 1976 "Race, achievement, and delinquency: a further look at delinquency in a birth
        cohort." American Journal of Sociology 82:379–387.
Jesness, C.F.
 1965 The Fricot Ranch Study. Sacramento, CA: California Youth Authority.
 1971a "Comparative effectiveness of two institutional treatment programs for delin-
        quents." Child Care Quarterly 1:119–130.
 1971b "The Preston typology study." Journal of Research in Crime and Delinquency
        8:38–52.
 1975 "Comparative effectiveness of behavior modification and transactional analysis
        programs for delinquents." Journal of Consulting and Clinical Psychology
        43:758–779.
Johnson, G., T. Bird, J.W. Little and S.L. Beville
 1981 Delinquency Prevention: Theories and Strategies. Washington, D.C.: Office of
        Juvenile Justice and Delinquency Prevention.
Johnson, R.E.
 1979 Juvenile Delinquency and Its Origins. Cambridge, England: Cambridge Univer-
        sity Press.
Kassebaum, G., D. Ward and D. Wilner
 1971 Prison Treatment and Parole Survival. New York: Wiley.
Kellam, S.G., T.D. Branch, C.H. Brown and G. Russell
 1981 "Why teenagers come for treatment: a 10-year prospective epidemiological
        study in Woodlawn." Journal of the American Academy of Child Psychiatry
        20:477–495.
Kelling, G.L., T. Pate, D. Dieckman and C.E. Brown
 1976 "The Kansas City preventive patrol experiment: a summary report." Pp.
        605–657 in G.V. Glass (ed.). Evaluation Studies Review Annual. Volume 1.
        Beverly Hills, CA: Sage.

Kelly, F.J. and D.J. Baer
   1971   "Physical challenge as a treatment for delinquency." Crime and Delinquency
          17:437–445.
Kelly, T.M.
   1983   "Status offenders can be different: a comparative study of delinquent careers."
          Crime and Delinquency 29:365–380.
Kent v. United States
   1966   383 U.S. 541.
Klein, M.W.
   1967   Juvenile Gangs in Context. Englewood Cliffs, NJ: Prentice-Hall.
   1979   "Deinstitutionalization and diversion of juvenile offenders: a litany of imped-
          iments." Pp. 145–201 in N. Morris and M. Tonry (eds.). Crime and Justice:
          An Annual Review of Research. Volume 1. Chicago: University of Chicago
          Press.
   1984   "Offense specialization and versatility among juveniles." British Journal of
          Criminology 24:185–194.
Knight, B.J., S.G. Osborn and D.J. West
   1977   "Early marriage and criminal tendency in males." British Journal of Criminol-
          ogy 17:348–360.
Knight, B.J. and D.J. West
   1975   "Temporary and continuing delinquency." British Journal of Criminology
          15:43–50.
Kobrin, S. and M.W. Klein
   1983   Community Treatment of Juvenile Offenders: The DSO Experiments. Beverly
          Hills, CA: Sage.
Krisberg, B. and I. Schwartz
   1983   "Rethinking juvenile justice." Crime and Delinquency 29:333–364.
Kumar, S.P., E.K. Anday, L.M. Sacks, R.Y. Ting and M. Delivoria-Papadopoulos
   1980   "Follow-up studies of very low birth weight infants (1250 grams or less) born and
          treated within a perinatal center." Pediatrics 66:438–444.
Lamb, H. and V. Goertzel
   1974   "Ellsworth House: a community alternative to jail." American Journal of Psy-
          chiatry 131:64–68.
Langan, P.A. and D.P. Farrington
   1983   "Two-track or one-track justice? some evidence from an English longitudinal
          survey." Journal of Criminal Law and Criminology 74:519–546.
Langner, T.S., J.C. Gersten and J.G. Eisenberg
   1977   "The epidemiology of mental disorder in children: implications for community
          psychiatry." Pp. 69–109 in G. Serban (ed.). New Trends of Psychiatry in the
          Community. Cambridge, MA: Ballinger.
Larson, R.C.
   1975   "What happened to patrol operations in Kansas City?" Journal of Criminal
          Justice 3:267–297.
Lee, R. and N.M. Haynes
   1980   "Project CREST and the dual treatment approach to delinquency: methods and
          research summarized." Pp. 169–184 in R.R. Ross and P. Gendreau (eds.). Effec-
          tive Correctional Treatment. Toronto: Butterworth.
Lefkowitz, M.M., L.D. Eron, L.O. Walder and L.R. Huesmann
   1977   Growing Up to be Violent. New York: Pergamon.

Lemert, E.M.
  1951   Social Pathology. New York: McGraw-Hill.
  1967   Human Deviance, Social Problems and Social Control. Englewood Cliffs, NJ: Prentice-Hall.
  1976   "Response to critics: feedback and choice." Pp. 244–249 in L.A. Coser and O.N. Larson (eds.). The Uses of Controversy in Sociology. New York: Free Press.
Lenihan, K.J.
  1977   Unlocking the Second Gate. Washington, D.C.: U.S. Government Printing Office.
Lerman, P.
  1975   Community Treatment and Social Control. Chicago: University of Chicago Press.
Lewis, R.V.
  1983   "Scared straight—California style." Criminal Justice and Behavior 10:209–226.
Lichtman, G.M. and S.M. Smock
  1981   "The effects of social service on probation recidivism: a field experiment." Journal of Research in Crime and Delinquency 18:81–100.
Liker, T.J.
  1982   "Wage and status effects of employment on affective well-being among ex-felons." American Sociological Review 47:264–283.
Lipton, D., R. Martinson and J. Wilks
  1975   The Effectiveness of Correctional Treatment: A Survey of Treatment Evaluation Studies. New York: Praeger.
Loeber, R.
  1982   "The stability of antisocial and delinquent child behavior: a review." Child Development 53:1431–1446.
Loeber, R. and T. Dishion
  1983   "Early predictors of male delinquency: a review." Psychological Bulletin 94:68–99.
  1984   "Boys who fight at home and school: family conditions influencing cross-setting consistency." Journal of Consulting and Clinical Psychology 52:759–768.
Loeber, R., T.J. Dishion and G.R. Patterson
  1984   "Multiple gating: a multistage assessment procedure for identifying youths at risk for delinquency." Journal of Research in Crime and Delinquency 21:7–32.
Lundman, R.J.
  1984   Prevention and Control of Juvenile Delinquency. New York: Oxford University Press.
Lundman, R.J., R.E. Sykes and J.P. Clark
  1978   "Police control of juveniles: a replication." Journal of Research in Crime and Delinquency 15:74–91.
Magnusson, D. and A. Duner
  1981   "Individual development and environment: a longitudinal study in Sweden." Pp. 111–122 in S.A. Mednick and A.E. Baert (eds.). Prospective Longitudinal Research. Oxford: Oxford University Press.
Magnusson, D., A. Duner and G. Zetterblom
  1975   Adjustment. Stockholm: Almqvist & Wiksell.
Maltz, M.D., A.C. Gordon, D. McDowall and R. McCleary
  1980   "An artifact in pretest–posttest designs: how it can mistakenly make delinquency programs look effective." Evaluation Review 4:225–240.

Martin, S.E., L.B. Sechrest and R. Redner (eds.)
   1981 New Directions in the Rehabilitation of Criminal Offenders. Washington, D.C.:
       National Academy Press.

Martinson, R.M.
   1974 "What works? questions and answers about prison reform." Public Interest
       35:22–54.

Matza, D.
   1964 Delinquency and Drift. New York: Wiley.

McCord, J.
   1977 "A comparative study of two generations of native Americans." Pp. 83–92 in
       R.F. Meier (ed.). Theory in Criminology. Beverly Hills, CA: Sage.
   1978 "A thirty-year follow-up of treatment effects." American Psychologist
       33:284–289.
   1979 "Some child-rearing antecedents of criminal behavior in adult men." Journal of
       Personality and Social Psychology 37:1477–1486.
   1982 "A longitudinal view of the relationship between paternal absence and crime."
       Pp. 113–128 in J. Gunn and D.P. Farrington (eds.). Abnormal Offenders, Delin-
       quency, and the Criminal Justice System. Chichester, England: Wiley.

McCord, W., J. McCord and I.K. Zola
   1959 Origins of Crime. New York: Columbia University Press.

McEwen, C.A.
   1978 Designing Correctional Organizations for Youth. Cambridge, MA: Ballinger.

McKee, G.J.
   1985 "Cost-benefit analysis of vocational training." Pp. 316–324 in R.M. Carter, D.
       Glaser and L.T. Wilkins (eds.). Correctional Institutions. Third edition. New
       York: Harper and Row.

McKeiver v. Pennsylvania
   1971 403 U.S. 528.
   1918 "The psychology of punitive justice." American Journal of Sociology
       23:577–602.

Mead, G.H.
   1934 Mind, Self and Society. Chicago: University of Chicago Press.

Mednick, S.A., W.F. Gabrielli and B. Hutchings
   1983 "Genetic influences in criminal behavior: evidence from an adoption cohort."
       Pp. 39–56 in K.T. Van Dusen and S.A. Mednick (eds.). Prospective studies of
       crime and delinquency. Boston: Kluwer-Nijhoff.

Mednick, S.A. and J. Volavka
   1980 "Biology and crime." Pp. 85–158 in N. Morris and M. Tonry (eds.). Crime and
       Justice: An Annual Review of Research. Volume 2. Chicago: University of
       Chicago Press.

Mennel, R.
   1973 Thorns and Thistles: Juvenile Delinquents in the United States, 1825–1940.
       Hanover, NH: University Press of New England.

Meyer, H.J., E.F. Borgatta and W.C. Jones
   1965 Girls at Vocational High. New York: Russell Sage.

Miller, A.D. and L.E. Ohlin
   1985 Delinquency and Community. Beverly Hills, CA: Sage.

Miller, F.J.W., S.D.M. Court, E.G. Knox and S. Brandon

1974 The School Years in Newcastle Upon Tyne. London: Oxford University Press.

Miller, M.O. and M. Gold
1984 "Iatrogenesis in the juvenile justice system." Youth and Society 16:83–111.

Miller, S.J., S. Dinitz and J.P. Conrad
1982 Careers of the Violent. Lexington, MA: Heath.

Miller, W.B.
1958 "Lower-class culture as a generating milieu of gang delinquency." Journal of Social Issues 14:5–19.
1962 "The impact of a 'total-community' delinquency control project." Social Problems 10:168–191.

Monahan, J.
1981 Predicting Violent Behavior: An Assessment of Clinical Techniques. Beverly Hills, CA: Sage.

Morash, M.
1982 "Juvenile reaction to labels: an experiment and an exploratory study." Sociology and Social Research 67:76–88.

Morris, N.
1974 The Future of Imprisonment. Chicago: University of Chicago Press.

Morris, P.
1965 Prisoners and Their Families. London: Allen and Unwin.
1975 On License: A Study of Parole. London: Wiley.

Mrad, D.F.
1979 "The effect of differential follow-up on rearrests: a critique of Quay and Love." Criminal Justice and Behavior 6:23–29.

Murray, C.A.
1983 "The physical environment and community control of crime." Pp. 107–122 in J.Q. Wilson (ed.). Crime and Public Policy. San Francisco: Institute for Contemporary Studies.

Murray, C.A. and L.A. Cox
1979 Beyond Probation: Juvenile Corrections and the Chronic Delinquent. Beverly Hills, CA: Sage.

O'Donnell, C.R., T. Lydgate and W.S.O. Fo
1979 "The buddy system: review and follow-up." Child Behavior Therapy 1:161–169.

Office of Juvenile Justice and Delinquency Prevention
1982 Delinquency Prevention: From Theory to Practice. Washington, D.C.: U.S. Department of Justice.

Ohlin, L.E.
1954 "The stability and validity of parole experience tables." Unpublished doctoral dissertation, University of Chicago.

Osborn, S.G. and D.J. West
1978 "The effectiveness of various predictors of criminal careers." Journal of Adolescence 1:101–117.
1980 "Do young delinquents really reform?" Journal of Adolescence 3:99–114.

Osbun, L. and P.A. Rode
1984 "Prosecuting juveniles as adults." Criminology 22:187–202.

Palmer, T.B.
1971 "California's community treatment program for delinquent adolescents." Journal of Research in Crime and Delinquency 8:74–92.

1974 "The youth authority's community treatment project." Federal Probation 38(1):3–14.

1978 Correctional Intervention and Research. Lexington, MA: D.C. Heath.

Pate, T., G.L. Kelling and C. Brown

1975 "A response to 'what happened to patrol operations in Kansas City?'" Journal of Criminal Justice 3:299–320.

Patterson, G.R.

1974 "Intervention for boys with conduct problems: multiple settings, treatment and criteria." Journal of Consulting and Clinical Psychology 43:471–481.

1980a "Children who steal." Pp. 73–90 in T. Hirschi and M. Gottfredson (eds.). Understanding Crime. Beverly Hills, CA: Sage.

1980b "Treatment for children with conduct problems: a review of outcome studies." Pp. 83–132 in S. Feshbach and A. Fraczek (eds.). Aggression and Behavior Change: Biological and Social Processes. New York: Praeger.

Patterson, G.R., P. Chamberlain and J.B. Reid

1982 "A comparative evaluation of a parent-training program." Behavior Therapy 13:638–650.

Peck, R.F. and R.J. Havighurst

1960 The Psychology of Character Development. New York: Wiley.

Petersilia, J. and P.W. Greenwood

1978 "Mandatory prison sentences: their projected effects on crime and prison populations." Journal of Criminal Law and Criminology 69:604–615.

Petersilia, J., P.W. Greenwood and M. Lavin

1978 Criminal Careers of Habitual Felons. Washington, D.C.: U.S. Department of Justice.

Peterson, M.A., H.B. Braiker and S.M. Polich

1981 Who Commits Crimes? Cambridge, MA: Oelgeschlager, Gunn, & Hain.

Piliavin, I. and S. Briar

1964 "Police encounters with juveniles." American Journal of Sociology 70:206–214.

Police Foundation

1981 The Newark Foot Patrol Experiment. Washington, D.C.: Police Foundation.

Polk, K., C. Alder, G. Bazemore, G. Blake, S. Cordray, G. Coventry, J. Galvin and M. Temple

1981 Becoming Adult: An Analysis of Maturational Development From Age 16 to 30 of a Cohort of Young Men. Eugene, OR: University of Oregon Department of Sociology.

Porporino, F.J. and E. Zamble

1984 "Coping with imprisonment." Canadian Journal of Criminology 26:403–421.

Powers, E. and H. Witmer

1951 An Experiment in the Prevention of Delinquency. New York: Columbia University Press.

President's Commission on Law Enforcement and Administration of Justice

1967 Task Force Report: Juvenile Delinquency and Youth Crime. Washington, D.C.: U.S. Government Printing Office.

Pritchard, D.

1979 "Stable predictors of recidivism: a summary." Criminology 17:15–21.

Quay, H.C.

1977 "The three faces of evaluation: what can be expected to work?" Criminal Justice and Behavior 4:341–354.

Quay, H.C. and C.T. Love

1977   "The effect of a juvenile diversion program on rearrests." Criminal Justice and
        Behavior 4:377–396.

1979   "Effects of a juvenile diversion program on rearrests: a reply to Mrad." Criminal
        Justice and Behavior 6:31–33.

Rankin, J.H. and L.E. Wells

1985   "From status to delinquent offenses: escalation?" Journal of Criminal Justice
        13:171–180.

Reckless, W.C. and S. Dinitz

1972   The Prevention of Juvenile Delinquency: An Experiment. Columbus, OH: Ohio
        State University Press.

Reimer, E. and M. Warren

1957   "Special intensive parole unit." National Probation and Parole Association Jour-
        nal 3:222–229.

Richards, B.

1978   "The experience of long-term imprisonment." British Journal of Criminology
        18:162–169.

Risman, B.J.

1980   "The Kansas City preventive patrol experiment: a continuing debate." Evalua-
        tion Review 4:802–808.

Robins, L.N.

1966   Deviant Children Grown Up. Baltimore, MD: Williams and Wilkins.

1978   "Aetiological implications in studies of childhood histories relating to antisocial
        personality." Pp. 255–271 in R.D. Hare and D. Schalling (eds.). Psychopathic
        Behavior. New York: Wiley.

1979   "Sturdy childhood predictors of adult outcomes: replications from longitudinal
        studies." Pp. 219–235 in J.E. Barrett, R.M. Rose and G.L. Klerman (eds.).
        Stress and Mental Disorder. New York: Raven Press.

Robins, L.N. and K.S. Ratcliff

1980   "Childhood conduct disorders and later arrest." Pp. 248–263 in L.N. Robins, P.J.
        Clayton and J.K. Wing (eds.). The Social Consequences of Psychiatric Illness.
        New York: Brunner/Mazel.

Robins, L.N., P.A. West and B.L. Herjanic

1975   "Arrests and delinquency in two generations: a study of black urban families and
        their children." Journal of Child Psychology and Psychiatry 16:125–140.

Robins, L.N. and E. Wish

1977   "Childhood deviance as a developmental process: a study of 223 urban black
        men from birth to 18." Social Forces 56:448–473.

Robinson, W.S.

1950   "Ecological correlations and the behavior of individuals." American Sociologi-
        cal Review 15:351–357.

Rojek, D.G. and M.L. Erickson

1982   "Delinquent careers." Criminology 20:5–28.

Rose, G. and R.A. Hamilton

1970   "Effects of a juvenile liaison scheme." British Journal of Criminology 10:2–20.

Ross, H.L.

1973   "Law, science, and accidents: the British road safety act of 1967." Journal of
        Legal Studies 4:1–78.

Ross, H.L., D.T. Campbell and G.V. Glass

1970   "Determining the social effects of a legal reform: the British 'breathalyser'
        crackdown of 1967." American Behavioral Scientist 13:493–509.

Ross, H.L., R. McCleary and T. Epperlein
  1982 "Deterrence of drinking and driving in France." Law and Society Review
        16:345-374.
Rossi, P.H., R.A. Berk and K.J. Lenihan
  1980 Money, Work, and Crime. New York: Academic Press.
  1982 "Saying it wrong with figures: a comment on Zeisel." American Journal of
        Sociology 88:390-393.
Ruhland, D.J., M. Gold and R.J. Hekman
  1982 "Deterring juvenile crime: age of jurisdiction." Youth and Society 13:353-376.
Rutter, M.
  1981 "Epidemiological/longitudinal strategies and causal research in child psy-
        chiatry." Journal of the American Academy of Child Psychiatry 20:513-544.
Rutter, M. and H. Giller
  1984 Juvenile Delinquency: Trends and Perspectives. New York: Guilford Press.
Rutter, M., B. Maughan, P. Mortimore and P. Ouston
  1979 Fifteen Thousand Hours: Secondary Schools and Their Effects on Children.
        Somerset, England: Open Books.
Sarason, I.G.
  1978 "A cognitive-social learning approach to juvenile delinquency." Pp. 299-317 in
        R.D. Hare and D. Schalling (eds.). Psychopathic Behavior: Approaches to
        Research. Chichester, England: Wiley.
Sarason, I.G. and V.J. Ganzer
  1973 "Modeling and group discussion in the rehabilitation of juvenile delinquents."
        Journal of Counseling Psychology 20:442-449.
Schlossman, S.
  1983 "Juvenile justice: history and philosophy." In. S.H. Kadish (ed.). Encyclopedia
        of Crime and Justice. New York: Free Press.
Schlossman, S. and M. Sedlak
  1983 "The Chicago area project revisited." Crime and Delinquency 29:398-462.
Schmid, C.F.
  1960 "Urban crime areas: part II." American Sociological Review 25:655-678.
Schneider, A.L.
  1984 "Divesting status offenses from juvenile court jurisdiction." Crime and Delin-
        quency 30:347-370.
Schnelle, J.F., R.E. Kirchner, J.D. Casey, P.H. Uselton and M.P. McNees
  1977 "Patrol evaluation research: a multiple-baseline analysis of saturation police
        patroling during day and night hours." Journal of Applied Behavior Analysis
        10:33-40.
Schnelle, J.F., R.E. Kirchner, F. Galbaugh, M. Domash, A. Carr and L. Larson
  1979 "Program evaluation research: an experimental cost-effectiveness analysis of an
        armed robbery intervention program." Journal of Applied Behavior Analysis
        12:615-623.
Schnelle, J.F., R.E. Kirchner, J.W. Macrae, M.P. McNees, R.H. Eck, S. Snodgrass, J.D.
    Casey and P.H. Uselton
  1978 "Police evaluation research: an experimental and cost-benefit analysis of a
        helicopter patrol in a high crime area." Journal of Applied Behavior Analysis
        11:11-21.
Schnelle, J.F., R.E. Kirchner, M.P. McNees and J.M. Lawler
  1975 "Social evaluation research: the evaluation of two police patroling strategies."
        Journal of Applied Behavior Analysis 8:353-365.

Schnelle, J.F. and J.F. Lee
1974 "A quasi-experimental retrospective evaluation of a prison policy change." Journal of Applied Behavior Analysis 7:483–496.

Schur, E.M.
1971 Labeling Deviant Behavior: Its Sociological Implications. New York: Harper and Row.

Schwartz, R.D. and S. Orleans
1967 "On legal sanctions." University of Chicago Law Review 34:274–300.

Schwartz, I.M., M. Jackson-Beeck and R. Anderson
1984 "The hidden system of juvenile control." Crime and Delinquency 30:371–385.

Schweinhart, L.J. and D.P. Weikart
1980 Young Children Grow Up: The Effects of the Perry Preschool Program on Youths Through Age 15. Ypsilanti, MI: High/Scope.

Sechrest, L. and R. Redner
1979 "Strength and integrity of treatments in evaluation studies." In How Well Does It Work? Washington, D.C.: National Institute of Law Enforcement and Criminal Justice.

Sechrest, L., S.O. White and E.D. Brown (eds.)
1979 The Rehabilitation of Criminal Offenders: Problems and Prospects. Washington, D.C.: National Academy of Sciences.

Severy, L.J. and J.M. Whitaker
1982 "Juvenile diversion: an experimental analysis of effectiveness." Evaluation Review 6:753–774.

Shah, S.A. and L.H. Roth
1974 "Biological and psychophysiological factors in criminality." Pp. 101–173 in D. Glaser (ed.). Handbook of Criminology. Chicago: Rand McNally.

Shannon, L.W.
1981 Assessing the Relationship of Adult Criminal Careers to Juvenile Careers. Iowa City, IA: Iowa Urban Community Research Center.

Shaw, M.
1974 Social Work in Prison. London: Her Majesty's Stationery Office.

Shaw, C.R. and H.D. McKay
1969 Juvenile Delinquency and Urban Areas. Revised edition. Chicago: University of Chicago Press.

Sheldon, W.H., E.M. Hartl and E. McDermott
1949 Varieties of Delinquent Youth. New York: Harper and Row.

Sherman, L.W.
1983 "Patrol strategies for police." Pp. 145–163 in J.Q. Wilson (ed.). Crime and Public Policy. San Francisco: Institute for Contemporary Studies.

Sherman, L.W. and R.A. Berk
1984 "The specific deterrent effects of arrest for domestic assault." American Sociological Review 49:261–272.

Shields, J.
1962 Monozygotic Twins Brought Up Apart and Brought Up Together. London: Oxford University Press.

Slavin, R.E.
1980 "Cooperative learning." Review of Educational Research 50:315–342.

Smith, R.L.
1983 (April) "Corrections: an update of the 1967 presidential task force report on

corrections." Unpublished report. Washington, D.C.: National Institute of Corrections.

Smith, C.F.W. and J.R. Hepburn
  1979 "Alienation in prison organizations: a comparative analysis." Criminology 17:251–262.

Spence, S.
  1982 "Social skills training with young offenders." Pp. 107–134 in P. Feldman (ed.). Developments in the Study of Criminal Behavior. Volume 1. Chichester, England: Wiley.

Stapleton, W.V. and L.E. Teitelbaum
  1972 In Defense of Youth. New York: Russell Sage.

Sutherland, E.H. and D.R. Cressey
  1969 "A sociological theory of criminal behavior." Pp. 426–432 in D.R. Cressey and D.A. Ward (eds.). Delinquency, Crime, and Social Process. New York: Harper and Row.
  1974 Criminology. Ninth edition. Philadelphia: Lippincott.

Sviridoff, M. and J.Q. Thompson
  1983 "Links between employment and crime: a qualitative study of Rikers Island releases." Crime and Delinquency 29:195–212.

Tannenbaum, F.
  1938 Crime and Community. Boston: Ginn.

Tarling, R.
  1982 "Unemployment and crime." Home Office Research Bulletin 14:28–33.

Telch, M.J., J.D. Killen, A.L. McAlister, C.L. Perry and N. Maccoby
  1982 "Long-term follow-up of a pilot project on smoking prevention with adolescents." Journal of Behavioral Medicine 5:1–8.

Thomas, C.W.
  1976 "Are status offenders really so different?" Crime and Delinquency 22:438–455.

Thomas, C.W. and D.M. Petersen
  1977 Prison Organization and Inmate Subcultures. Indianapolis, IN: Bobbs-Merrill.

Thornberry, T.P. and M. Farnworth
  1982 "Social correlates of criminal involvement: further evidence on the relationship between social status and criminal behavior." American Sociological Review 47:505–518.

Tittle, C.R.
  1980a Sanctions and Social Deviance. New York: Praeger.
  1980b "Labelling and crime: an empirical evaluation." Pp. 241–263 in W.R. Gove (ed.). The Labelling of Deviance: Evaluating a Perspective. Second edition. Beverly Hills, CA: Sage.

Toby, J.
  1983a "Violence in school." Pp. 1–47 in M. Tonry and N. Morris (eds.). Crime and Justice: An Annual Review of Research. Volume 4. Chicago: University of Chicago Press.
  1983b "Crime in the schools." Pp. 69–88 in J.Q. Wilson (ed.). Crime and Public Policy. San Francisco: Institute for Contemporary Studies.

Toch, H.
  1975 Men in Crisis: Human Breakdowns in Prison. Chicago: Aldine.
  1977 Living in Prison: The Ecology of Survival. New York: Free Press.

Tornudd, P.
  1968 "The preventive effect of fines for drunkenness." Pp. 109–124 in N. Christie (ed.). Scandinavian Studies in Criminology. Volume 2. London: Tavistock.

Trasler, G.B.
  1962 The Explanation of Criminality. London: Routledge and Kegan Paul.

Vaillant, G.E.
  1983 The Natural History of Alcoholism. Cambridge, MA: Harvard University Press.

Van Dine, S., J.P. Conrad and S. Dinitz
  1979 Restraining the Wicked. Lexington, MA: Heath.

Van Dusen, K.T. and S.A. Mednick
  1983 A Comparison of Delinquency in Copenhagen and Philadelphia. Final Report to the National Institute of Justice. Washington, D.C.: National Institute of Justice.

Venezia, P.S.
  1972 "Unofficial probation: an evaluation of its effectiveness." Journal of Research in Crime and Delinquency 9:149–170.

Vosburgh, W.W. and L.B. Alexander
  1980 "Long-term follow-up as program evaluation: lessons from McCord's 30-year follow-up of the Cambridge–Sommerville youth study." American Journal of Orthopsychiatry 50:109–124.

Wadsworth, M.E.J.
  1976 "Delinquency, pulse rates, and early emotional deprivation." British Journal of Criminology 16:245–256.
  1979 Roots of Delinquency. London: Robertson.

Waldo, G.P. and T.A. Chiricos
  1977 "Work release and recidivism: an empirical evaluation of a social policy." Evaluation Quarterly 1:87–108.

Walker, N.
  1980 Punishment, Danger, and Stigma. Oxford: Blackwell.

Waller, I.
  1974 Men Released from Prison. Toronto: University of Toronto Press.

Weis, J.G., R. Janvier and J.D. Hawkins
  1981 Overview of Delinquency Prevention Research and Development Project. Seattle, WA: Center for Law and Justice, University of Washington.

Wellford, C.F.
  1973 "Age composition and the increase in recorded crime." Criminology 11:61–70.
  1975 "Labeling theory and criminality: an assessment." Social Problems 22:332–345.

Werner, E.E. and R.S. Smith
  1982 Vulnerable but Invincible. New York: McGraw-Hill.

West, D.J.
  1982 Delinquency: Its Roots, Careers, and Prospects. London: Heinemann.

West, D.J. and D.P. Farrington
  1973 Who Becomes Delinquent? London: Heinemann.
  1977 The Delinquent Way of Life. London: Heinemann.

Wheeler, S.
  1961 "Socialization in correctional instructions." American Sociological Review 26:697–712.

Wiatrowski, M.D., D.B. Griswold and M.K. Roberts
1981 "Social control theory and delinquency." American Sociological Review 46:525–541.
Williams, M.
1970 A Study of Some Aspects of Borstal Allocation. London: Home Office Prison Department, Office of the Chief Psychologist.
1975 "Aspects of the psychology of imprisonment." Pp. 32–42 in S. McConville (ed.). The Use of Imprisonment. London: Routledge and Kegan Paul.
Wilson, H.
1980 "Parental supervision: a neglected aspect of delinquency." British Journal of Criminology 20:203–235.
Wilson, J.Q.
1980 "'What works?' revisited: new findings on criminal rehabilitation." Public Interest 61:3–17.
1983 (October) "Raising kids." Atlantic Monthly 45–56.
Wilson, J.Q. and R.J. Herrnstein
1985 Crime and Human Nature. New York: Simon and Schuster.
Wilson, J.Q. and G.L. Kelling
1982 (March) "Broken windows." Atlantic Monthly 29–38.
Wirt, R.D. and P.F. Briggs
1959 "Personality and environmental factors in the development of delinquency." Psychological Monographs 73(15): No. 485.
Witkin, H.A., S.A. Mednick, F. Schulsinger, et al.
1976 "Criminality in XYY and XXY men." Science 193:547–555.
Wolf, P.
1984 "Delinquent boys and family relations." In P. Wolf (ed.). Sequential Research. Volume 1. Copenhagen: Micro Publications Social Science Series.
Wolfgang, M.E.
1974 "Crime in a birth cohort." Pp. 79–92 in R. Hood (ed.). Crime, Criminology, and Public Policy. London: Heinemann.
1980 "Some new findings from the longitudinal study of crime." Australian Journal of Forensic Sciences 13:12–29.
1983 "Delinquency in two birth cohorts." Pp. 7–16 in K.T. Van Dusen and S.A. Mednick (eds.). Prospective Studies of Crime and Delinquency. Boston: Kluwer-Nijhoff.
Wolfgang, M.E., R.M. Figlio and T. Sellin
1972 Delinquency in a Birth Cohort. Chicago: University of Chicago Press.
Wolfgang, M.E. and P.E. Tracy
1982 (February) "The 1945 and 1958 birth cohorts: a comparison of the prevalence, incidence, and severity of delinquent behavior." Paper presented at conference on "Public Danger, Dangerous Offenders, and the Criminal Justice System," Harvard University, Cambridge, MA.
Zeisel, H.
1982a "Disagreement over the evaluation of a controlled experiment." American Journal of Sociology 88:378–389.
1982b "Hans Zeisel concludes the debate." American Journal of Sociology 88:394–396.

Zimring, F.E.
　1981　"Kids, groups, and crime: some implications of a well-known secret." Journal of
　　　　Criminal Law and Criminology 72:867–885.
Zimring, F.E. and J.G. Hawkins
　1973　Deterrence: The Legal Threat to Crime Control. Chicago: University of Chicago
　　　　Press.

Author Index

Subject Index